RADIOSENSITIZERS OF HYPOXIC CELLS

To Professor Pietro Bucalossi one of the Italian pioneers of cancer research and treatment.

RADIOSENSITIZERS OF HYPOXIC CELLS

Editors

A. Breccia
C. Rimondi

and

G.E. Adams

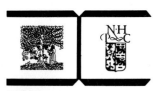

1979

ELSEVIER/NORTH-HOLLAND BIOMEDICAL PRESS
AMSTERDAM · NEW YORK · OXFORD

ISBN Elsevier/North-Holland: 0-444-80124-3

Published by:
Elsevier/North-Holland Biomedical Press
335 Jan van Galenstraat, P.O. Box 211
Amsterdam, The Netherlands

Sole distributors for the USA and Canada:
Elsevier North-Holland Inc.
52 Vanderbilt Avenue
New York, N.Y. 10017

Library of Congress Cataloging in Publication Data
Main entry under title:

Radiosensitizers of hypoxic cells.

    "Based on the summer course 'Mechanism of action of
radiosensitizers of hypoxic cells in vitro and in
vivo' held in Cesenatico August 21 to September 1, 1978."
    Bibliography: p.
    1. Cancer--Radiotherapy--Congresses. 2. Radiation
-sensitizing agents--Congresses. 3. Cells, Effect of
drugs on--Congresses. 4. Anoxemia--Congresses.
I. Breccia, A. II. Rimondi, C. III. Adams, G. E.
[DNLM: 1. Anoxia--Congresses. 2. Radiation-sensitizing agents--Pharmacodynamics--Congresses. WN610.3
R129 1978]

RC271.R3R335   611'.0181   79-10617
ISBN 0-444-80124-3

Printed in The Netherlands

PREFACE

The present volume is based on the summer course "Mechanism of action of radiosensitizers of hypoxic cells *in vitro* and *in vivo*" held in Cesenatico August 21 to September 1, 1978.

The work includes not only the texts of the fifteen seminars that were held in Cesenatico, but also the results of laboratory experiments carried out in Bologna. Distinguished scientists from both Italy and Europe have contributed extensive reviews of several extremely relevant and significant subjects, that will be of great interest to clinicians and researchers throughout the world.

The organizers of the course, Professors A. Breccia, C. Rimondi and G.E. Adams, succeeded in emphasizing the relevance of a phenomenon already recognised as very important in other countries, namely, the clinical applicability of drugs capable of magnifying radiation therapy effects. Indeed, the volume reflects the hope that the achievement of an increase in the radiosensitivity of highly resistant tumors might not be too distant.

The course was held under the patronage of the Lega Italiana per la lotta contro i tumori (Italian league for the fight against tumors) following the wishes of P. Breccia, who has now asked me to present this work to a wider scientific audience. I certainly hope that the publication of this volume will achieve this aim.

G.F. GARDINI

Presidente della Sezione bolognese della
Lega Italiana per la lotta contro i tumori

CONTRIBUTORS

ADAMS G.E.
- Physics Division, Institute of Cancer Research, Clifton Avenue, Sutton, Surrey, England.

BADIELLO R.
- Laboratorio di Fotochimica e Radiazioni di Alta Energia, CNR, Via Castagnoli 3, Bologna.

BRECCIA A.
- Cattedra di Chimica Generale, Università di Bologna, Via Zanolini,3,Bologna.

BUSI F.
- Laboratorio di Fotochimica e Radiazioni di Alta Energia, CNR, Via Castagnoli,3, Bologna.

DISCHE S.
- Radiotherapy Div., Mount Vernon Hospital, Northwood, Middlesex.

FOWLER J.F.
- Gray Laboratory, Mount Vernon Hospital, Northwood, Middlesex.

GATTAVECCHIA E.
- Facoltà di Farmacia, Università di Bologna, Via Selmi,2, Bologna.

PRODI G.
- Istituto di Cancerologia, Università di Bologna, Via S. Giacomo, Bologna.

RIMONDI C.
- Divisione di Radioterapia, Ospedale Malpighi, Via P.Pelagi, Bologna.

ROFFIA S.
- Istituto Chimico G.Ciamician, Università di Bologna, Via Selmi,2, Bologna.

STRATFORD I.J.
- Physics Division, Institute of Cancer Research, Clifton Avenue, Sutton, Surrey, England.

TAMBA M.
- Laboratorio di Fotochimica e Radiazioni di Alta Energia, CNR, Via Castagnoli, 3, Bologna.

WARDMAN P.
- Molecular Biology, Gray Laboratory, Mount Vernon Hospital, Northwood, Middlesex.

INTRODUCTION

For many years, radiotherapists and radiobiologists have shown an increasing interest in the development and clinical application of radiosensitizing drugs for hypoxic cells.

This prompted us to organize an advanced teaching course, at a postgraduate level, embracing physical, chemical, biological and clinical aspects of the field.

The course included the following subjects:
- correlation between the chemical and structural properties of radiosensitizing drugs with their biological activity
- pharmaco-kinetic properties of radiosensitizers, in biochemical and biological systems as studied by polarographic, chromatographic, spectrophotometric and radiochemical methods
- cellular aspects of sensitization *in vitro* and *in vivo*
- clinical studies with hypoxic cell sensitizers.

The course comprised of fifteen lectures and two days of experimentation using pulse radiolysis and electrochemical techniques. The lectures were given at the University Center for Marine Biology and Sea Productivity, Cesenatico, Italy and the experimental projects were carried out in the Institute of Chemistry, University of Bologna and in the Laboratory of Radiation Chemistry, C.N.R., Bologna, Italy.

The Organizers gratefully acknowledge the generous financial support and the granted fellowships for the participants to:

Lega Italiana per la Lotta Contro i Tumori;

Ospedale "Malpighi" di Bologna;

Azienda Autonoma de Soggiorno e Turismo di Cesenatico;

Camera de Commercio, Industria, Agricoltura de Forlì;

Istituto De Angeli de Milano;

Rotary Club di Cervia e Cesenatico;

Ministero per la Pubblica Istruzione;

Consorzio per il Centro Universitario di Biologia Marina, Cesenatico.

Special thanks are due to the Lega Italiana per la Lotta Contro i Tumori, sezione di Bologna and the Società Cesenate corse al trotto under whose auspices and support the course was organized.

A. Breccia
C. Rimondi
G.E. Adams

CONTENTS

© 1979 Elsevier/North-Holland Biomedical Press
Radiosensitizers of Hypoxic Cells
A. Breccia, C. Rimondi and G.E. Adams eds.

CONCEPTS OF RADIOSENSITIZATION AND TECHNIQUES OF INVESTIGATION

A. BRECCIA

Cattedra di Chimica Generale e Inorganica, Facoltã di Farmacia - Università
di Bologna, Bologna, Italy.

1) GENERAL

Radiosensitization is the process whereby the effects of ionizing
radiations are enhanced by chemical agents.

The classification of these chemical agents follows two criteria. One is
based upon their effects at a biological level:

1) suppression of compounds containing SH groups or of other radioprotectors;

2) formation of radiation-induced   cytotoxic products;

3) DNA incorporation of thymine analogues;

4) inhibition of cellular regrowth.

The other criteria concern chemical or physical properties of the compounds
such as their electron affinity or oxygen mimicy.

Effects of the radiosensitizing chemical agents have been known for
many years but a systematic study of the mechanism of action of all types
of radiosensitization in general has developed only during the last five years[1]
and still many aspects of the phenomenon are to be clarified.

Even the mechanism of action of hypoxic cell sensitizers, which has been
suggested by Adams as early as 1963[2] is still not completely clear. Hower
current knowledge of the behaviour of electron affinic drugs enables us to
apply them in human radiotherapy.

The present paper is concerned with the physico-chemical principles of
the mechanism of action of the electron affinic compounds, and the techniques
used to study them.

2) CRITERIA FOR INVESTIGATING THE PHYSICO-CHEMICAL MECHANISM OF SENSITIZATION

Electrons, as well as OH and H radicals are the most abundant products of
the radiolysis process of biological tissues since water is the largest

constituent of the cellular mass, (about 80-85%). Therefore water is the most effective absorber of energy and its products of radiolysis participate in the reactions occurring inside the irradiated cell. In hypoxic cells, hydrated electrons as well as bio-radicals or bio-ions are presumably produced and therefore the electron affinic properties of sensitizing drugs would appear to be the most important from the point of view of both reactions with polarized molecules and of electron transfer reactions.

If we look at the electron reaction mechanism the electron may react with two species A and B in aqueous solution as follows:

$$A + e_{aq}^{-} \xrightarrow{k_1} A^{-}$$

$$B + e_{aq}^{-} \xrightarrow{k_2} B^{-}$$

The reactions of the two compounds are characterized by rate constants $k_1(A)$ and $k_2(B)$ respectively.

If however, the two reactants differ in their electron affinities, an electron transfer reaction can occur:

$$A^{-} + B \longrightarrow B^{-} + A \qquad \text{or}$$

$$A + B^{-} \longrightarrow A^{-} + B$$

Other more complicated electron transfer reactions are known to occur also in living systems. An example in a chemical system could be the chain transfer reaction of different ketones in alkaline solution[3]:

acetone + e_{aq}^{-} $\longrightarrow$ acetone^{-} $\longrightarrow$ acetophenone^{-} $\longrightarrow$ benzophenone^{-} $\longrightarrow$ p. nitrobenzophenone^{-}.

From these kinetic observations one can surmise that the rate constants of the reactions with the electrons are ultimately responsible for the radiosensitizing properties of the test molecules.

Table 1 collects the values of rate constants for reaction of hydrated electrons with various compounds, which have lifetimes in the range of microseconds or less[4].

TABLE 1

Compounds	Velocity constant of e^-_{aq} reaction
	$k \ (M^{-1} \ s^{-1})$
p. nitrotoluene	1.9×10^{10}
Nitrobenzene	3.0×10^{10}
Picric Ac.	3.9×10^{10}
O_2	2.0×10^{10}
DNA	$- \ 10^{12}$
Metronidazole	2.2×10^{10}
DA 3827	1.8×10^{10}
Imidazole	3.7×10^{7}
DA 3838	2.6×10^{10}
Piridine	1.0×10^{9}
Adenosine	3.0×10^{10}

Since reactions with electrons are extremely fast and the decay times of the transient species produced are very short, fast response techniques are necessary to study their mechanisms at a molecular level, e.g. pulse radiolysis, kinetic spectrophotometry or rapid-mixing.

3) THE IRRADIATION AND THE BIOLOGICAL MECHANISM OF SENSITIZATION

In a living system during irradiation there are different stages of the radiolysis process extending from the physico-chemical primary steps to the biological repair or degradation processes. This is shown in fig. 1[5].

The processes studied at the physico-chemical stage are very fast as explained above and they consist of molecular excitation and of ion and radical formation. At this stage, the biomolecules irradiated are still in polar conditions. Further reactions proceed through two fundamental biological stages with radiation induced products or with other compounds present in the living systems[6]; for example:

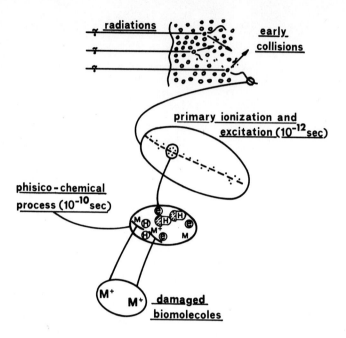

Fig. 1 - Radiation-tissue interaction

1) molecular degradation,

$$R' + O_2 \longrightarrow RO_2'$$

2) molecular repair,

$$R' + -SH \longrightarrow RH + -S^{\cdot}$$

The probability that one of the two processes occur depends on the kinetics of the two reactions. In the example given the oxygen reaction is faster than the other and it is favoured on kinetic grounds.

The mechanism of molecular damage is at the base of the action of the hypoxic cell sensitizers even if it is not yet clear whether it is the same for the oxygen mimics and electron affinic compounds. For the latter type Adams as previously mentioned[2] suggested a scheme in which electron transfer processes of the compounds are fundamental to their mechanism of action:

$$\text{biotargets} \xrightarrow[\text{irradiation}]{\text{hr}} \overset{+}{\wedge\wedge\wedge}\overset{-}{} \xrightarrow[\text{electron}]{\text{RS}} \text{RS}^- + \overset{\cdot\;\;+}{\wedge\wedge\wedge\vee} \longrightarrow$$
$$\text{transfer}$$

$$\longrightarrow \overset{\cdot\;\;\;+}{\wedge\wedge\wedge\vee}$$
$$\text{damaged}$$
$$\text{biomolecules}$$

Preliminary electrochemical studies[7] seem to provide evidence of another process where by the hydrated, or free, electrons react with the radiosensitizer outside the cell, C, and then are transferred to the cell, inside or at the surface of the cell membranes:

$$RS + e^- \longrightarrow RS^-$$

$$RS^- + C \longrightarrow C^- + RS$$

Cell molecules possibly involved in these two kinds of electron reaction are respectively the phosphoglycidic groups of DNA inside the cell and the polar groups of phospholipidic membrane outside the cell[8]. In both cases there is a good correlation between the electron affinity of the compounds and their radiosensitizing properties[9].

This correlation is expressed in Table 2 by the monoelectron redox potentials of the compounds referred to a concentration giving an Enhancement Ratio of 1.6. The term ENHANCEMENT RATIO, or ER, represents the increased efficiency of radiation in the presence of chemical agents with respect to the effect of radiation alone.

Some of the more interesting molecules tested as radiosensitizers *in vitro* and *in vivo* are listed in Table 3. It must be noted that only two compounds have been studied in clinical radiotherapy: metronidazole and misonidazole. They are generally nitroderivatives of aromatic or heterocyclic compounds.

The mono electron redox potentials is related to the $-NO_2$ group and is affected by the N-5 and C-5 side chains. The redox thereshold potential under which sensitization does not occur corresponds presumably to the redox potentials of the reacting bioradicals. Over that threshold potential the hypoxic cell killing occurs exponentially unil an E.R. value equal to that of Oxygen is reached.

TABLE 2

Compounds	Substituents at N-5	Substituents at C-5	Monoelectron redox potential at pH = 7	Sensitizer concentration for ER = 1.6 (mmol dm^{-1})
L 8711	CH_3	CHO	- 243	0.02
L 7138	$CH_2CO_2CH_2CH_3$	CH_3CH_2	- 388	0.35
Ro-05-9963	$CH_2CH(OH)CH_2OH$	H	- 389	0.9
Ro-07-0582	$CH_2CH(OH)CH_2OCH_3$	H	- 389	0.3
Ro-07-0554	CH_2CH_2OH	H	- 398	0.3
L 6802	$CH_2CH_2OCOCH_3$	CH_3	- 420	1.0
L 6678	CH_2CH_2OH	CH_3	- 423	1.0
Metronida-zole	CH_2CH_2OH	CH_3	- 486	4

This chemical radiosensitization indicates a controlled redox relationship between bioradicals and sensitizers in competition with other radical reactions.

4) THE TECHNIQUES FOR THE STUDY OF HYPOXIC CELL RADIOSENSITIZING

The mono electron redox potential, E_7', has been determined[10] by the measurement of the equilibrium constant, K, of the reaction $ArNO_2^- + Q \longrightarrow$ $\longrightarrow ArNO_2 + Q^-$, where Q is a redox reference compound such as Quinone and Q^- is its radical ion. The $ArNO_2^-$ and Q^- are generally unstable in water solutions at pH 7, so the K must be measured by means of a fast response technique such as pulse radiolysis.

Another method of measuring E_7' is to apply cyclic voltammetry[11]. The graph is fig. 2 shows a comparison of monoelectron peak redox potential, E_{pc}', measured by electrochemical methods with the E_7' measured by the pulse radiolysis technique. In the case of utilization of the cyclic voltammetry the limits of the used apparatus are due to the time response which cannot be shortes than m sec.

TABLE 3

Formulae				Symbols

Nitro-imidazoles derivatives	Substituent at			
	C-5	N-1	C-2	
	- CHO	$-CH_2$		L 8711
2-Nitro	$-CH(OCOCH_3)_2$	$-CH_3$		L 10926
	-H	$-CH_2CHOHCH_2OCH_3$		Ro-07-0582 (misonidazole)
4-Nitro	-Cl	$-CH_3$	-H	B
	-H	-H	-H	I
				DA 3829
5-Nitro	Compounds not yet registered			DA 3831
				DA 3837
	H	$-CH_2-CH_2OH$		J
	$-CH_2CH_2OH$	$-CH_3$		Flagyl (metronidazole)

Other Nitroderivatives

NDPP (Roche), p.nitro-3-dimethylamino-propriophenone. HCl

MTDQ, 6,6'-methylen, bis 2,2,4-trimethyl-1,2-dihydroquinoneline

Nifurpipone (Recordati), 5-nitro-2-furfuraldehyde-N'-methyl-N-piperazon-
        acetonidrazone, diclorohydrate

p-nitrobenzyl alcool	A
nitrofurenone	E
m-nitroacetophenone	G
p-nitroacetophenone	
nitrofuroxime	H

Quinone

duroquinone	F

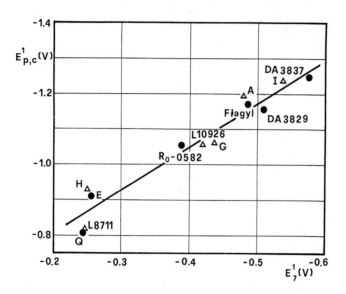

Fig. 2 - Peak potential E'_{pc} for the first cathodic process, against one-
-electron potentials E'_7 from pulse radiolysis.

The ● and △ symbols in the Figure indicate the reversibility and non-
reversibility of the electron reactions with the compounds. The symbols
of the compounds are explained in Table 3.

It is not yet clarified as to role the reversibility of electron
reactions play in the mechanism of action of the different radiosensitizers.
However, it must be pointed out that the use of electrochemical methods
appears to be very promising with regard to the many kinds of problems
concerning the mechanism of action of hypoxic cell sensitizers. Indeed
these techniques are complementary to pulse radiolysis.

In particular, the polarographic technique is useful for studying:
- electron reactions occurring at the surface of cell membranes;
- the various reduction steps of the nitrocompounds and of other electron
  affinic molecules and the influence of reduced derivatives on cell
  sensitization;
- the penetration of radiolabelled sensitizers into cells;
- the concentration of drugs and of their metabolites in the blood.

Cyclic voltammetry on the other hand could be utilized to study:

- the reversibility of electron reactions of the drugs under investigation;

- the catalytic processes of electron transfer reactions with the drugs.

In preliminary experiments many of these processes have been examined and first results are very promising[7].

More informations will be given in a subsequent paper by Roffia and Co-workers.

The polarographic technique provides also a fast method for determining the blood level of metronidazole and misonidazole in patients[12].

5) CELL SENSITIZATION INVESTIGATION

At the cell level, the basic information necessary to understand the mechanism of action of hypoxic cell sensitizers is their cytoxic properties, and their concentration inside tumour cells.

Cytoxicity of sensitizers must be evaluated before testing for sensitization. Account must be taken of any toxicity due to the radiation-induced formation of toxic substances.

The concentration of drug inside cells or tissues is generally measured indirectly from the blood concentration of the drug. It is believed that the level of the compounds in the cell is of the same order as that present in the blood[12].

The survival curve and the factors affecting cell killing during irradiation can be represented from the Zimmer equation[13] $S = (1 - e^{-D/D_o})^m$ where Do is the main lethal dose, D is the irradiation dose and m is the multitarget species. In fig. 3 a typical survival curve is shown.

As already shown data of this type are a fundamental prerequisite to the assessment of the E.R. of any new drugs and therefore to their application in preclinical and clinical studies.

Also for the mechanism of the action of these cell sensitizers, it is very important to know the influence of the cell toxicity, concentration in the tumour tissue, kinetics of the cell after treatment with sensitizers, and the formation of their metabolites as we will see in forthcoming papers.

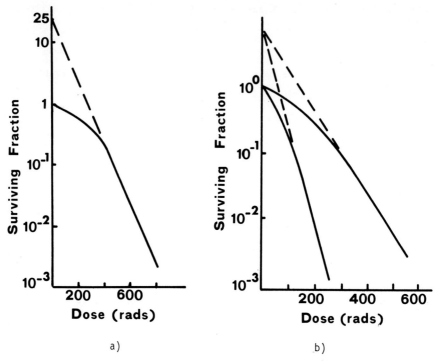

a)   b)

Fig. 3 - % of surviving fraction, a) with X-rays only; b) with X-ray and sensitizers.

REFERENCES

1. Philips, T.L., Cancer, 39, 987, 1977.

2. Adams, G.E., and Dewey, D.L., (1963) Biochem.Biophys.Res.Comm.12:473.

3. Badiello, R., Breccia, A., Chim. Ind., 1976, 57, 525.

4. Anber, M., Neta, P., Int. J. Rad. Isot., 18, 493, 1967.

5. Breccia, A., Convegno C.N.R. su Fotochimica e Chimica radiazioni, 1975, 141, Ed. C.N.R.

6. Adams, G.E., Agnew, D.A., I.J. Stratford and Wardman, P., Proceed. V Symp. Microdosimetry, 1975, p. 17.

7. Breccia, A., Roffia, S., Gattavecchia, E., work in progress, 1978.

8. Biaglow, J.E., Greenstock, C.L., Durand, R.E., Brit. J. Cancer, 37, 1978, Suppl. III, 145.

9. Fowler, J.F., Adams, G.E., and Denekamp, J.,Cancer treatment Reviews, 1976, 3, 227.

10. Wardman, P., and Clarke, E.D., (1976) J. Chem. Soc. Faraday Trans. I, 72, 1377.

11. Breccia, A., Roffia, S., Berrilli, G., Int. Jour. of Rad. Biol., in press, 1979.

12. Dische, S., Saunders, M.I., Lee, M.E., Adams, G.E., and Flockart, I.R., Br. J. Cancer, 35, 567, 1977.

13. Zimmer, K.G., (1961), "Quantitative radiation biology" Oliver, R., Boyd, Edimburghs.

Radiosensitizers of Hypoxic Cells
A. Breccia, C. Rimondi and G.E. Adams eds.

PROSPECTS AND PROBLEMS WITH HYPOXIC CELL RADIATION SENSITIZERS

G.E. ADAMS

Physics Division, Institute of Cancer Research, Clifton Avenue, Sutton, Surrey, England, SM2 5PX.

INTRODUCTION

The fundamental objective in the clinical use of ionizing radiation to sterilize human tumours is to give the maximum possible radiation dose to the tumour while at the same time keeping as low as possible, the radiation dose unavoidably delivered to normal tissues surrounding the tumour. Developments in radiotherapy physics have done much towards achieving this goal. In the area of tumour localisation, techniques such as isotope scanning, diagnostic ultrasound and the rapidly - expanding use of computerised axial tomography (CAT scanning) have all contributed to better treatment planning. Methods of delivering a high radiation dose to the tumour while sparing as much as possible, surrounding normal tissue have also improved considerably following the introduction of mega-voltage irradiation machines during the decade following the second world war.

However, at the present time, notwithstanding the very advanced treatment methods available, failure of local tumour control by radiotherapy is still a problem - in some sites particularly so. Even though metastasis remains a major problem in cancer therapy, failure to eradicate the disease locally is responsible for a significant proportion of cancer mortality. Even when treated with the maximum possible radiation doses, some human tumours only respond partially and ultimately regrow. There are probably several reasons for this but with little doubt, a major cause for local failure is the problem of the hypoxic cell.

There is now very good evidence that hypoxic cells, i.e. cells which at the time of radiation, are very low in oxygen content, occur in significant proportion of human tumours. Hypoxic cells arise as a result of tumour growth

14

essentially out-stripping its blood supply. They occur usually in and around
areas of necrosis which are often seen in micro-histological preparations
of both animal and human tumours.

The accepted model for hypoxic cells in tumours is that proposed by
Thomlinson and Gray based on their histological examinations of rat tumours.[1]
Their model is illustrated in figure 1.

THOMLINSON-GRAY MODEL

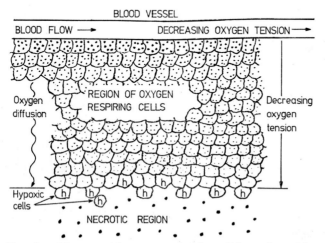

Fig. 1 - Diagrammatic representation of hypoxic cell model.

Viable cells lining, and near to, a micro-capillary in a tumour are fairly
well oxygenated by the oxygen delivered to the tumour by the blood supply.
Division can occur provided the oxygen tension is sufficient for the
requirements of the cell. However, the oxygen tension decreases radially
outwards from the capillary and eventually falls below the level required
to sustain potential viability. Cells sufficiently remote from a blood vessel,
die, and this is the reason for the necrotic areas usually seen occurring at
a distance of about 150-200 microns from the blood vessel. Hypoxic cells are
believed to occur in the interface region between the viable tumour tissue
and the necrotic areas.

Why are these hypoxic cells dangerous? They are dangerous because relative
to the oxygenated cell, they are resistant to radiation. Hypoxic cell

radioresistance is a well-known universal phenomenon in radiobiology, observed in virtually all bacteria, plant cells and mammalian cells of widely-differing types. Hypoxic cells are in a resting state and of course, would eventually die. However; following treatment of a tumour by radiation, regression occurs, due to the removal of oxic cells sterilized by the radiation. This permits some of the hypoxic cells to be re-oxygenated. They enter cycle, divide and provide therefore, a focus for the regrowth of the tumour.

THE MAGNITUDE OF THE OXYGEN EFFECT

In general, the cellular response to radiation-killing is an exponential function of radiation dose although in mammalian cells and some bacteria, the exponential region of the survival curve is usually preceded by a short shoulder region.

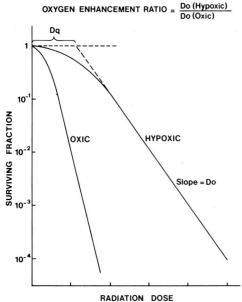

$$\text{OXYGEN ENHANCEMENT RATIO} = \frac{Do\,(Hypoxic)}{Do\,(Oxic)}$$

Fig. 2 - Representation by survival curves of the differente radiation sensitivities of oxic and hypoxic cells.

The radiation sensitivity is defined as the slope of the linear portion of the semi-logarithmic plot of the surviving fraction (D_o). In mammalian cells, the oxygen enhancement ratio (OER), defined as the ratio of the D_o

values for hypoxic and oxic cells is usually about 3 and relatively small amounts of oxygen are required to manifest the effect. In respiring cells in most normal tissue, the oxygen supply is adequate for the radiation sensitivity to be at, or near, the maximum level. In tumours, most of the malignant respiring cells will also be sufficiently oxygenated to be radiation sensitive. However, the influence of the presence of even a very small proportion of hypoxic cells on the overall radiation sensitivity of a tumour is indicated diagrammatically in figure 3.

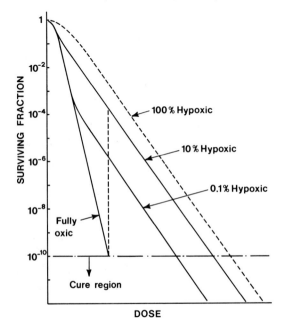

Fig. 3 - Theoretical single,-dose survival cells for a population of 10^{10} cells containing different proportions of hypoxic cells (See text).

Let us consider theoretically the total radiation doses required to sterilise a tumour containing about 10^{10} viable cells of which, say 10% and 0.1% are hypoxic. Also suppose it is necessary to sterilise all of the cells by radiation. The response of the hypoxic and oxic cells to a *single* dose of radiation would be expected to follow the survival curves shown in the figure depending upon the fraction of hypoxic cells. At very low doses, the response of the more numerous oxic cells predominates. However, the dose is soon attained where the majority of the surviving cells are hypoxic and ultimately at the dose level required to sterilize all the oxic cells, there is still a significant surviving fraction of hypoxic cells (indicated by the vertical dotted line). It is apparent, that even if the *initial* hypoxic fractions were even lower, some hypoxic cells would still survive a radiation dose sufficient to kill all the oxic cells.

In actual radiotherapy practice, tumours are of course not treated by single doses of radiation, but are treated rather with a course of multiple small doses given over several weeks. Clinical experience has long since shown that such fractionated treatments give much better results. There are several likely reasons for this, the discussion of which is outside the scope of this lecture. However, one likely contributory factor to the better results obtained with fractionated ratiation is the phenomenon of *re-oxygenation*.

In some experimental animal tumour systems, it has been shown conclusively that if the time schedule for the radiation fractionation is appropiate, some hypoxic cells can be re-oxygenated during the intervals between the radiation fractions. This means that the total number of hypoxic cells surviving a complete course of fractionated radiation could be considerably less than would survive if re-oxygenation did not occur.

Without doubt, re-oxygenation must play some rôle in the overall response of human tumours to fractionated radiotherapy and may well be the major reason why some tumours respond exceedingly well. However, tumours can vary widely in re-oxygenation efficiency and some may re-oxygenate hardly at all during treatment. Those human tumours that respond badly to radiotherapy are probably the ones that either re-oxygenate poorly - if at all - or do so over a time scale different to that of the fractionation schedules usually given in the clinic.

METHODS OF OVERCOMING THE HYPOXIC CELL PROBLEM

At present, there are four methods available for attempting to eliminate or considerably reduce the number of hypoxic cells present in tumours. They are the following.

a) Unconventional fractionation

Over the years, various clincial trials have been carried out using unconventional fractionation regimes. While such studies have been essentially empirical in design and not necessarily directed solely at the hypoxia problem, any significant influence of radiation scheduling on the proportion of hypoxic cells present in tumours could theoretically result in a change in the radiation sensitivity of those tumours. To date, however, little has been learned concerning the influence of fractionation on the hypoxia status of human tumours. Because of the wide variability of human tumours in their radiation response, it would be surprising indeed if fraction scheduling *alone*, could achieve total elimination of the hypoxic problem in human tumours.

b) Treatment in hyperbaric oxygen

A more promising approach to the hypoxia problem followed the pioneering work of Churchill-Davidson and others on the use of high pressure oxygen tanks in radiotherapy[2]. During the last twenty years, various trials have taken place in which patients have been given radiotherapy while lying in a specially-constructed pressure vessel. This permits the patients to breathe up to 3 atmospheres pressure of oxygen during the course of each radiation treatment. The rationale behind this technique is that the increased concentration of free oxygen in the blood should result in a considerable increase in the range of oxygen diffusion from a tumour capillary. Hypoxic cells beyond the normal range of oxygen diffusion would be oxygenated and thus could be rendered radiation sensitive.

Numerous clinical trials with this technique have been carried out over the years. Some have indeed indicated a margin of benefit to the patients. However, there are serious disadvantages with hyperbaric oxygen. The technique is not without some risk to the patient, it requires specialised apparatus and above all is extremely demanding on the time and resources of the radiotherapy clinic. As is discussed later, it is by no means certain that breathing hyperbaric oxygen permits oxygenation of *all* of the hypoxic cells in the tumour.

c) Heavy particle radiotherapy

Elsewhere in this lecture series, Dr. Fowler discusses the application of heavy particle radiation in radiotherapy. There are several reasons behind this approach; one is concerned with the hypoxia problem. It has long been recognised in experimental radiobiology that the magnitude of the oxygen effect decreases with the increasing 'LET' of the radiation. Linear Energy Transfer (LET) is a measure of the rate at which energy is deposited in a material irradiated with ionizing radiation. For densely-ionizing radiations, such as high energy neutrons, the fall in the OER means that the relative protective effect of hypoxia is reduced. With neutron irradiation hypoxic cells are still, more radiation-resistant than oxic cells, but *relatively* much less so compared with X- or electron irradiation.

Clinical trials of neutron radiotherapy are in progress and hopefully will demonstrate improved results. However, the fact remains, that at present such methods are expensive, requiring as they do, specialised treatment machines. Further, while the oxygen effect is considerably reduced with high LET radiotherapy, it is *not* completely eliminated.

d) Chemical sensitizers for hypoxic cells

In principle, the use of chemical drugs which *specifically* increase the radiation sensitivity of hypoxic cells would be the preferred method of overcoming the hypoxia problem. They would be cheap, and if free of complications, could be used routinely in radiotherapy without the need to invest in expensive apparatus or treatment machines, and would not necessitate any increase in the work-load.

There are now many chemical compounds which specifically sensitize hypoxic cells in vitro and some of these are active *in vivo* also. However, for virtually all hypoxic cell sensitizers, their efficiencies, defined in terms of the concentrations required for a given degree of sensitization, are less than that of oxygen. One might ask therefore why should such drugs offer any advantage over the use of hyperbaric oxygen?

A vital difference between the principle of action of hypoxic cell sensitizers and that of oxygen, is that provided the sensitizers are not

rapidly metabolised by the tumour tissue through with they diffuse, they
will penetrate further than oxygen and thus be able to reach all the hypoxic
cells in the tumour. Figure 4 illustrates schematically this fundamental
difference in principle.

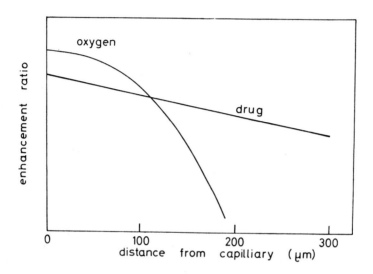

Fig. 4 - Theoretical representation of the sensitizing ratios for oxygen
and drug for cells at various distances from a nearest capillary.

The diagram shows how the enhancement ratio for sensitization of hypoxic
cells is affected by the distance between these cells and the nearest blood
vessel. For the oxygen curve, sensitization disappears at about 200 microns
distance. An increased oxygen supply in the blood vessel caused by
breathing hyper-baric oxygen will extend the diffusion distance but there
is still likely to be a steep oxygen gradient. In contrast, a sensitizer
than in concentration terms in *less efficient* than oxygen, will be a *more
effective* sensitizer in the regions of the tumour with a poor blood supply:
provided the drug is not rapidly metabolised.

THE DEVELOPMENT OF HYPOXIC CELL SENSITIZERS

The generality of the oxygen effect in radiobiology has for many years stimulated the search for chemical compounds that produce the same effect. At the present time there are many such agents known, all of which show sensitization of hypoxic cells but have no effect on oxic cells. By far the largest class of such sensitizers is the "Electron-affinic group", so called because the efficiency of sensitization defined in terms of the concentrations required to produce a given degree of sensitization, is related to the electron-affinities or the reduction potentials of the compounds[3,4,5,6].

The electron affinity proposal led to the examination of many different types of chemical structures for evidence of radiation-sensitizing properties. In the early years test systems used were generally micro-organisms including various strains of bacteria[7] and bacterial spores[8]. Compounds found to possess sensitizing ability included quinones, various other conjugate diketones, aromatic ketones, diesters and other miscellaneous molecules all containing conjugate electron-accepting groups in their structure.

While much evidence was accumulating for sensitization of hypoxic micro--organisms by these compounds, little information was forthcoming on sensitization of hypoxic *mammalian* cells - even in systems *in vitro*. Some of the stable nitroxyl free-radicals such as tri-acetoneamine-N-oxyl were found to exhibit some sensitization of hypoxic Chinese Hamster cells in vitro[9,10]. However these compounds, which are not members of the electron-affinic group, are metabolically unstable and are virtually inactive *in vivo*.

However, shortly after the results with the nitroxyls were reported, it was found that the electron-affinic sensitizer para-nitroacetophenone (PNAP) showed appreciable sensitization of hypoxic Chinese Hamster cells *in vitro*[11,12]. No sensitization occurred in the presence of oxygen and it was found that the efficiency of sensitization showed little variation with the position of the cell in the mitotic cycle[12]. Unfortunately, the very low solubility of PNAP greatly restricted attempts to demonstrate sensitization of hypoxic cells *in vivo* although slight sensitization was reported using a soluble derivative of PNAP in an experimental mouse tumour system[13].

About this time, Chapman and colleagues reported that various nitrofurans showed considerable sensitization of hypoxic mammalian cells *in vitro*[14]. This was significant because some of the nitrofurans tested were already in clincial use as anti-bacterial agents particularly in urinary infections. However, subsequent attempts to demonstrate sensitization *in vivo* with these compounds has been generally disappointing since the nitrofurans appear to be toxic at the dose levels required for sensitization.

At the present time, relatively few compounds show appreciable sensitization *in vivo*. Undoubtedly, this is due mainly to the difficulties in penetrating into the regions of tumours where hypoxic cells occur. Clearly, for a sensitizer to be effective *in vivo*, it must be sufficiently metabolically stable to enable it to diffuse intra-cellularly to the hypoxic cells which are probably situated 150-200 microns from the nearest capillary.

Fortunately, a range of compounds are now known whose metabolic stabilities are satisfactory in this respect. In 1973 it was reported that the 5-nitroimidazole Metronidazole or "Flagyl" was able to sensitize both hypoxic bacteria and mammalian cells[14,15]. Although this compound is

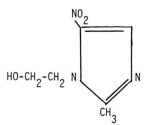

Metronidazole

relatively inefficient an a concentration basis, its half-life in vivo is fairly long. Various experiments showed significant sensitization of the response of mouse tumours to irradiation. A comprehensive account of the various methods used to measure sensitization *in vivo* with metronidazole and other hypoxic cell sensitizers in presented by Dr. Fowler elsewhere in these proceedings.

Misonidazole

The successes with Metronidazole led to the search for more active compounds the nitroimidazole series. In this lecture course Dr. Wardman and Dr. Badiello discuss the chemical basis for the development of hypoxic cell sensitizers generally and the molecular models for the study of their mechanism of action. Only a brief comment is necessary therefore on the reason underlying the development of sensitizers more active than Metronidazole.

Considerations of the electron affinity relationship led naturally to the proposition that the substituted 2-nitroimidazoles would be better sensitizers. This was based on the expectation that a nitro group substituted in the 2-position of the imidazole ring would interact to a greater degree with the π-electron system, of the heterocyclic ring than would a nitro group substituted in the 5-position. On examination of a range of 2-nitroimidazoles originally synthesised by Roche Products, one such compound Ro-07-0582 or, as it is now termed misonidazole, was found to be a very efficient sensitizer both *in vitro* and *in vivo* [16,17].

Misonidazole

Figure 5 illustrates the sensitizing effect of misonidazole in Chinese Hamster cells irradiated *in vitro* in the presence of the drug. In oxygen, misonidazole has no effect on the cellular radiation response. However in nitrogen, the sensitization at 1 mM is marked and at a concentration of 10 mM the enhancement ratio is comparable to that of oxygen itself. Other studies *in vitro* showed that the efficiency of sensitization of misonidazole does not vary significantly with the position of the cell in the mitotic cycle [16].

The high sensitization efficiency of misonidazole in mammalian cells irradiated *in vitro* led to numerous studies of the drug as a sensitizer of experimental animal tumours. Data on the sensitization by misonidazole is

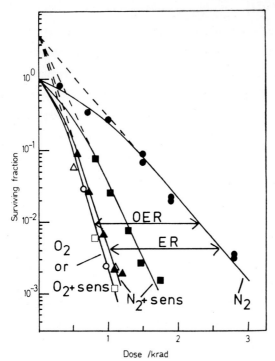

Fig. 5 - Survival data for hypoxic Chinese hamster V379A cells irradiated
in vitro with x-rays in the presence of 1 mmol. ■ and 10 mmol.
▲ of misonidazole. Data from reference 16.

certainly impressive (see Fowler, these proceedings). Enhancement ratios
of 2 or greater have been observed in a large number of experimental tumour
systems treated with single doses of radiation and sensitization is also
observed with multi-fraction irradiation.

CRITERIA FOR SENSITIZERS IN CLINICAL USE

The evidence accumulated from the large amount of experimental data from
the laboratory naturally led to consideration of pilot clinical studies of
misonidazole as a radiation sensitizer in man. Some of the main criteria
that would have to be satisfied for a radiation sensitizer to be useful
clinically are as follows:

a) Differential sensitization of tumour tissue only

Any drug that sensitized the radiation response of normal and malignant tissue to the same extent would be of little value. Misonidazole and other electron-affinic sensitizers are active only in hypoxia. Normal tissues which are generally well-oxygenated should not show any sensitization and this has been the clinical experience so far (see Dische - these proceedings). As is discussed by Fowler, there may be special circumstances where a small proportion of hypoxic cells occur in normal tissue. Such tissues might be at risk with large radiation doses but are unlikely to be so with multiple small fractions.

b) Low toxicity to normal tissues

Both metronidazole and misonidazole are both well tolerated in fairly high doses. Whether this will be so far other nitroimidazoles, however, remains to be seen. As is discussed later, clinical dosage of misonidazole is ultimately limited by a peripheral neuropathy. Present recommendations are that the total dose should not exceed 12g/m^2 [18]. Extensive studies of the uptake of misonidazole in human tumours have shown that, despite this dose limitation, the tumour levels should be associated with considerable sensitization. The fractionation scheme with which the drug is used will affect however the degree of sensitization.

c) Penetration of large tumours

Because of the often poor blood supply in large human tumours, drug penetrability is one of the common problems encountered in developing new chemotherapeutic agents. This is particularly true in the hypoxic cell sensitizer field since the target cells usually lie in the remote poorly--vascularized regions of tumours. In the past, numerous prototype sensitizers which have appeared to be extremely active *in vitro*, have proved to have little or no activity *in vivo*.

The nitromidazoles are exceptional in this respect. Tumour penetration, particularly with misonidazole does not appear to be a major problem, although in mice, the fairly short half-life in serum ($\sim$1 hour) coupled with fairly long diffusion time in tumours results in drug-tumour levels rarely exceeding about 30-40% of blood levels. However, in man where the serum half-life is 12 hours, tumour levels approaching blood levels are quite common.

Experience generally with misonidazole strongly indicates that the development of future drugs must take into account the need for considerable metabolic stability. Drug half-lives of at least several hours will almost certainly be necessary.

d) Sensitization with respect to position in the mitotic cycle

Cells which become hypoxic must eventually cease to progress through the mitotic cycle, until of course, they subsequently become re-oxygenated. Because of the oxygen requirement for the cellular biochemistry occurring during the cycle, it is likely that hypoxic cells are arrested fairly early on in the cycle, possibly at the G_1 - S boundary. If this is so, sensitizers that act only during the later stages of the cycle would be clearly of little value in radiotherapy. Effort has been devoted to the investigation of any cell-cycle dependence of the efficiencies of the electron-affinic drugs.

Chapman and colleagues used synchronized cultures of Chinese Hamster cells to show that the efficiency of PNAP was essentially maintained throughout the cell cycle[11]. Subsequently, their findings were confirmed with other electron affinic sensitizers including the nitrofurans, and in particular, misonidazole itself[15]. Significantly also, other *in vitro* studies have shown that misonidazole retains its efficiency irrespective of whether asynchronous cells are made hypoxic during either the log phase of culture growth or in plateau phase.

It is fairly reasonable to conclude therefore, that the sensitizing efficiencies of the electron-affinic sensitizers generally are not very dependent on the biochemical status of the hypoxic cell. However, it should be stressed that studies of this type must remain an essential part of the development of any new drug for ultimate clinical use.

e) Sensitization with multiple small doses

Obviously in view of current radiotherapy practice, it is essential that sensitization of hypoxic cells occurs with multi-fraction radiotherapy - even with those regimens employing quite small fraction sizes. Various *in vitro* studies have shown fairly conclusively that sensitization of hypoxic mammalian cells by misonidazole occurs at very low doses (<200 rad) and ought to occur therefore during the low dose fractions of conventional radiotherapy. It is significant in this respect that, in a recent co-operative clinical trial of hyperbaric oxygen, carried out under the aegis of the Medical Research Council (UK), statistically-significant benefit was recorded even though the radiotherapy was given in multiple fractions of about 200 rads per fraction.

Although sensitization could be influenced considerably by the extent of re-oxygenation occurring between treatment fractions, and hypoxic cells that are not re-oxygenated will still be sensitized by misonidazole even if the value of the dose per fraction is small.

PROSPECTS FOR MISONIDAZOLE

The vast amount of radiobiological and pharmacological data on sensitization with misonidazole is certainly impressive. Large sensitization factors are observed in a wide range of experimental animal tumour types and the drug levels measured in numerous human tumours are quite high.

Nevertheless, the human dosage of misonidazole is limited ultimately by its neurotoxicity and it is clear that this will prevent the drug from being used at a level necessary for the maximum degree of sensitization theoretically possible i.e. the full value of the oxygen enhancement ratio.

Figure 6 shows the enhancement ratio for sensitization of hypoxic Chinese Hamster cells as a function of the concentration in the medium. The proposition that such a curve might apply to sensitization of human tumours rests on two main assumptions.

1) The sensitization efficiency of misonidazole is not reduced for hypoxic cells *in vivo* compared to those *in vitro*.

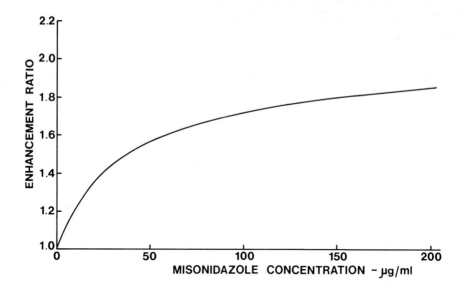

Fig. 6 - The enhancement ratios for sensitization of hypoxic Chinese hamster cells *in vitro* as a function of the concentration of misonidazole in the medium. Data from reference 16.

2) The concentration of the drug achieved in hypoxic tumour cells approaches that measured in the serum.

Both these assumptions appear to be justifiable at the present time. It has been shown in mouse tumours that the sensitizing efficiency of misonidazole *expressed relative to the drug concentration in the tumours* is at least as high as that measured *in vitro*. Further as indicated earlier, the rapidly increasing amount of data on drug penetration in human tumours shows that tumour levels are usually high and mostly at, or near, the levels measured in the serum.

It is recommended that the total clinical dose of misonidazole should not exceed $12g/m^2$ irrespective of the radiation fractionation scheme. Clearly therefore, the amount of drug per fraction will depend on the total number of fractions. This reasoning suggests that because of the total dose limitation, more benefit might be obtained with unconventional fractionation regimes using a relatively small number of large fraction sizes. This is one direction to pursue in clinical trials. However the implication of another property of sensitizer of this type - that of differential hypoxic cytotoxicity must be taken into account. This is discussed in a subsequent lecture which also deals with the prospects for developing other sensitizers more active than misonidazole.

REFERENCES

1. Thomlinson, R.H. and Gray, L.H. (1955) Brit. J. Cancer, 9, 539.

2. Churchill-Davidson, E., Sanger, C. and Thomlinson, R.H. (1955) Lancet, 10, 91.

3. Adams, G.E. and Dewey, D.L. (1963) Biochem. Biophys. Res. Commun., 12, 473.

4. Raleigh, J.A., Chapman, J.D., Borsa, J., Kremer, S.W. and Reuvers, A.P. (1973) Int. J. Radiat. Biol., 23, 377.

5. Simic, M. and Powers, E.L. (1974) Int. J. Radiat. Biol., 26, 87.

6. Adams, G.E., Flockhart, I.R., Smithen, C.E., Stratford, I.J., Wardman, P. and Watts, M.E. (1976) Radiat. Res., 67, 9.

7. Adams, G.E. and Cooke, M.S. (1969) Int. J. Radiat. Biol., 15, 457.

8. Tallentire, A., Schiller, M.L. and Powers, E.L. (1968) Int. J. Radiat. Biol., 14, 397.

9. Parker, L., Skarsgaard, L.D. and Emmerson, P.T. (1969) Radiat. Res., 38, 493.

10. Cooke, B.C., Fielden, E.M. and Johnson, M. (1976) Radiat. Res., 65, 152.

11. Adams, G.E., Asquith, J.C., Dewey, D.L., Foster, J.L., Michael, B.D. and Willson, R.L. (1971) Int. J. Radiat. Biol., 19, 575.

12. Chapman, J.D., Webb, R.G. and Borsa, J. (1971) Int. J. Radiat. Biol., 19, 561.

13. Sheldon, P.W. and Smith, A.M. (1975) Brit. J. Cancer, 31, 81.

14. Chapman, J.D., Reuvers, A.P., Borsa, J. Petkau, A. and McCalla, D.R. (1972) Cancer Res., 32, 2630.

15. Foster, J.L. and Willson, R.L. (1973) Brit. J. Radiol., 6, 234.

16. Asquith, J.C., Watts, M.E., Pattel, K.B., Smithen, C.E. and Adams, G.E. (L974) Radiat. Res., 60, 108.

17. For summary see Fowler (these Proceedings).
18. For summary see Dische(these Proceedings).

© 1979 Elsevier/North-Holland Biomedical Press
Radiosensitizers of Hypoxic Cells
A. Breccia, C. Rimondi and G.E. Adams eds.

A BRIEF SURVEY OF POLAROGRAPHY, LINEAR SWEEP VOLTAMMETRY, POTENTIAL CONTROLLED
ELECTROLYSIS AND COULOMETRY: UTILIZATION OF THESE TECHNIQUES IN THE STUDY OF
PROBLEMS INVOLVED WITH CHEMICAL RADIOSENSITIZATION OF HYPOXIC CELLS

SERGIO ROFFIA
Centro di Studio di Elettrochimica Teorica e Preparativa
Istituto Chimico "G. Ciamician", Università di Bologna (Italy)

INTRODUCTION

The following presentation is intended to familiarize non-electrochemists
with physico-chemical techniques which can be succesfully used in the field
of biological and medical research.

Many phenomena taking place in biological systems, such as energy transfer
processes, are frequently associated with electron transfer processes. Since
electrochemical techniques indicated in the title can give information both
on the thermodynamics and on the kinetics of redox reactions; it follows
that they are valuable for the investigation of biological systems.

In the present exposition, after the introduction of some basic definitions
and concepts of electrode kinetics, a brief illustration will be given of
the techniques indicated above, which are the most commonly used in the
study of electrode mechanisms. Finally,the results of the investigation
recently undertaken in our Institute for clarifying some aspects of the
chemical radiosensitization of hypoxic cells will be discussed.

BASIC CONCEPTS AND DEFINITIONS

Electrochemical systems

Electrochemical systems are characterized by an in series sequence of
first⁻kind conductors, such as metals and semiconductors, and second_kind
conductors, such as aqueous or non-aqueous solutions of electrolytes, molten
salts and solid electrolytes. The two first-kind conductors placed at either
end of the system are called *electrodes*, while the conductor sandwiched

between them is called *electrolyte*. If at one electrode a given electrochemical reaction results in a transfer of negative charges from the electrode to the solution, the associated current is called *cathodic*. If the opposite transfer occurs the current is called *anodic*. Thus one has *reductions* at the cathode and *oxidations* at the *anode* respectively.

Electrode processes

When current flows through an electrode,various modifications occur in the system associated with processes that allow the current flow. All such processes are termed *electrode process*. For example, in the case where a single reaction can take place at an electrode, the electrode process can be schematized thus:

1) transport of reagents from the bulk of the solution to the electrode surface;
2) homogeneous or heterogeneous chemical reactions giving rise to the chemical species subject to electron transfer;
3) charge transfer with electrons going from the electrode to the chemical species in the case of a cathodic process and vice-versa for a case of an anodic process;
4) homogeneous or heterogeneous chemical reactions involving the product of electron transfer;
5) transfer of the products into the bulk of the solution.

Electrochemical kinetics deal not only with the study of the electrochemical reaction proper, i.e. the charge transfer processes at the interface, but also with other phenomena involved in the electrode process such as mass transport and chemical reactions in with reagents or electron transfer products are implied.

Electrode potential

In the field of electrochemical kinetics the *electrode potential* is defined in a generalized sense as the difference of electrical potential between two identical metallic wires, one connected with the indicator electrode, the other connected with the reference electrode, ohmic drops being neglected.

The hydrogen electrode in standard conditions called the *normal hydrogen electrode* (NHE) is generally taken as a reference electrode, which is arbitrarily taken to have a potential of zero. Since the NHE is rather inconvenient for routine use it is common practice to measure electrode potentials with respect to a more easily handled reference electrode and of known potential with respect to NHE. In particular the *saturated calomel electrode* (SCE) is the most commonly used. Since SCE has a potential equal to 0.244 V against NHE at 25°C, all electrode potentials can be converted from the NHE scale to the SCE scale by adding 0.244 V.

Electrode polarization and overvoltage

When a current flows through an electrolytic cell the potentials of both electrodes are shifted by a variable amounts with respect to the value in the absence of current. This phenomena is called *electrode polarisation*. When only one reaction takes place at a given electrode, one defines *overvoltage* η as the difference between the electrode potential corresponding to a given current density E_i and the equilibrium potential E_e (or E_{rev}), which applies to currentless conditions $\eta = E_i - E_e$. E_e is a constant quantity for a given solution and for a given electrode reaction. The overall situation is schematized in Fig. 1 for a case of an electrolizer[*] , in which ohmic drops in the various phases are negligible. The terms $E_{i,a}$ and $E_{i,c}$ are referred to the electrode potentials of the anode and cathode respectively for a current density equal to i and by analogy, η_a and η_c are referred to the corresponding overvoltages. As it appears in this case, the overvoltage acts in the sense of increasing, with respect to the reversible values, the potential of the anode and of decreasing the potential of the cathode.

The source of polarization phenomena lies in the low rate of some partial process within the overall electrode process. If indeed an intrinsically slow step practically consumes all the energy available for dissipation, thus leaving all preceeding and following steps in very near-equilibrium

---

[*] An electrolizer is an electrochemical system where one has transformation of electric energy into chemical energy and heat.

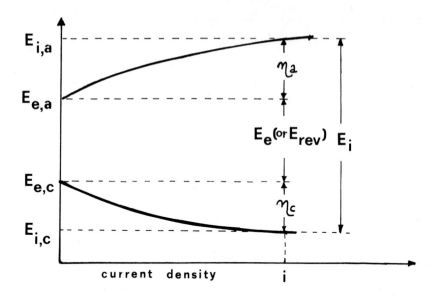

Fig. 1 - Potential - density current curves for an electrolizer.

conditions, this step by itself determines the velocity of the electrode
process. Such step is called the *rate determining step* and governs the
magnitude and type of total overvoltage η . According to the nature of the
rate determining step, which could be diffusion, charge transfer, chemical
reaction, an electrode process can be classified as diffusion controlled,
activation controlled, reaction controlled, etc. If two or more steps have
comparable velocities, they are shifted to a large extent from equilibrium
conditions and the overall overvoltage is the sum of the overvoltages resulting
from the individual slow processes. *A mixed kinetic control* results.

The determination of the *electrode potential* as a function of *current
density* results in plots that are called *polarization curves*. The recording
of polarization curves constitutes the basic method for the study of electrode
kinetics. Indeed the shape of polarization curves and their dependence on
solution composition, temperature, and on other physico-chemical parameters
allows us to gain detailed information on the nature of the electrode process.

Determination of Electrode Potentials. Three electrode assembly

When an electric potential difference E_i is applied to an electrochemical system, so that current i flows through the cell, the difference between the electrical potentials of electrodes 1,2 is given by:

$$E_i = E_{i,1} - E_{i,2} + \Delta V_\Omega = E_{i,1} - E_{i,2} + iR$$

where ΔV_Ω is the ohmic drop in the cell due to the resistance of the electrolyte, $E_{i,1}$ and $E_{i,2}$ are the electrode potentials as previously defined. In the above expression, ohmic drops in the electrodes are neglected. It might be pointed out that for kinetics investigations what matters are the electrode potentials, $E_{i,1}$ and $E_{i,2}$ and not the overall electrode potential difference E_i. Also, when studying the electrode mechanism, generally only one of the two electrodes in the cell is investigated. In view of these considerations a three electrode configuration is commonly used for the determination of the electrode potential. The cell current flows between the *working electrode* and the *counter electrode*, while the potential of the working electrode is measured with respect to the *reference electrode* using a high impedance measuring device. The reference electrode is connected to the cell via a salt bridge in order to minimize liquid junction potential, and via a Luggin-Haber capillary placed as close as possible to the working electrode. With the three electrode assembly the polarization of the reference electrode is avoided and the major portion of the iR drop in the cell is compensated.

Electron transfer kinetics. Reversible and irreversible processes

In discussing various types of polarization curves it is useful to briefly examine the fundamental laws regulating electron transfer kinetics. The case where only two steps contribute to the electrode process, i.e. mass transport by diffusion and electron transfer, will be considered. It will be assumed that the mass transfer takes place very rapidly, leaving electron transfer as the slow rate determining step. The electron transfer can be so schematized:

$$0 + ne \xrightleftharpoons[k_{b,h}]{k_{f,h}} R \tag{1}$$

The net current i is the difference between the current i_c associated with the reduction process (cathodic current) and the current i_a associated with the oxidation process (anodic current). In the present context cathodic currents are taken by convention to be positive and anodic currents negative:

$$i = i_c + i_a \tag{2}$$

where

$$i_c = nFAk_{f,h}C_O^\circ \qquad \text{and} \qquad i_a = -nFAk_{b,h}C_R^\circ \tag{3}$$

In (3) F stands for 96500 coulombs (1 Faraday), A is the electrode surface area, C_O° and C_R° are the concentrations of O and R at the electrode surface. The rate constants $k_{f,h}$ and $k_{b,h}$ characterize the kinetics of the electron transfer process and since they are associated with an heterogeneous process their dimensions are $1t^{-1}$. They also incorporate the activity coefficients of species O and R. The potential dependence of $k_{f,h}$ and $k_{b,h}$ is of exponential form according to the relations:

$$k_{f,h} = k_{f,h}^{ref} \exp \left[- \alpha nf(E - E_{ref}) \right] \tag{4}$$

$$k_{b,h} = k_{b,h}^{ref} \exp \left[(1-\alpha)nf(E - E_{ref}) \right] \tag{5}$$

where E is the potential determined with respect to a reference electrode potential E_{ref}, f = F/RT with R universal gas constant and T absolute temperature and α is the electron transfer coefficient[*]. Several such reference potentials are in use. If the reference potential of the NHE, which is null by definition, is utilized, one obtains:

---

[*] The values of α range from 0 to 1 and are generally close to 0.5. Experimentally it has often been found to be constant for a given electrode reaction over a wide range of electrode potentials.

$$k_{f,h} = k^\circ_{f,h} \exp(-\alpha nfE) \qquad \text{and} \qquad k_{b,h} = k^\circ_{b,h} \exp\left[(1-\alpha)nfE\right]$$

giving for i the following expression:

$$i = nFA \left\{ C^\circ_0 k^\circ_{f,h} \exp\left[(-nfE)\right] - C^\circ_R k^\circ_{b,h} \exp\left[(1-)nfE\right] \right\}$$

For $E = E_e$, $i = 0$, therefore

$$E_e = (1/nf)\left[\ln(k^\circ_{f,h}/k^\circ_{b,h}) + \ln(C^\circ_0/C^\circ_R)\right] = (1/nf)\left[\ln(k^\circ_{f,h}/k^\circ_{b,h}) + \ln(C^*_0/C^*_R)\right] \quad (6)$$

where C^*_0 and C^*_R are the bulk concentrations, and they coincide with C°_0 and C°_R respectively, since for $i = 0$ no concentration polarization is present. This equation corresponds to the Nernst equation for E°, standard potential, given by:

$$E^\circ = (1/nf)\ln(k^\circ_{f,h}/k^\circ_{b,h}) + (1/nf)\ln(f_R/f_0) \qquad (7)$$

where the f's are activity coefficients. The first term in the HRS of (7) is called the formal standard potential E°_c and represents the value assumed by the equilibrium potential when $C^*_0 = C^*_R$ (see Eq. 6)[*]. The latter can also be used as another reference potential. In this case, defining $k_{s,h}$ the common value of the rate constant for electron transfer for the forward and reverse process at potential E°_c, it is easy to show that:

$$i = nFAk_{s,h} \left\{ C^\circ_0 \exp\left[-\alpha nf(E-E^\circ_c)\right] - C^\circ_R \exp\left[(1-\alpha)nf(E-E^\circ_c)\right] \right\} \qquad (8)$$

The advantage of using E°_c as reference potential lies in the fact that only one rate constant, $k_{s,h}$ characterizes both cathodic process and anodic process:

$$i_c = nFAC^\circ_0 k_{s,h} \exp\left[-\alpha nf(E-E^\circ_c)\right] \qquad (9)$$

and

---

[*] The value of E°_c is generally not very different from the standard potential E° and can therefore often be identified with it.

$$i_a = -nFAC_R^\circ k_{s,h} \; exp \; \underline{/} \; (1-\alpha)nF(E-E_c^\circ) \underline{/} \qquad (10)$$

In order to understand the practical implication of terms such as *reversible* and *irreversible process*, the behaviour of two systems having equal formal standard potentials, but different values of $k_{s,h}$, can be examined. If the potential of the working electrode were to be suddenly varied with respect to the equilibrium potential, and the concentrations C_O° and C_R° were then monitored, one would find the following. Current would flow through the electrode so as to bring about, via the modifications described, a new equilibrium situation. If C_O° and C_R° do not reach equilibrium values before their determination at time t is effected, the potential will differ from the value calculated from the Nernst equation. The rate with which equilibrium values are reached will depend upon the size of i_c and i_a, which are in turn dependent on $k_{s,h}$. If the latter value is sufficiently high, the system will reach equilibrium within the experiment time scale, otherwise, it will not. In the first case the process is said to be reversible, in the second irreversible. For a reversible process, then, the potential can always be expressed in terms of the Nernst equation, even in cases of thermodynamically non-equilibrium situations, such as is the case where current flow occurs. Furthermore, from the description given above it appears evident that a given process, which under given conditions appears reversible, can become irreversible if the experimental time scale is reduced.

POLAROGRAPHY

Among various electrochemical techniques utilized for the study of redox reactions, polarography (P) plays a paramount role not only because of the simplicity of its instrumentation and for some fortunate experimental features associated with it, but also for providing the impulse toward the discovery of new electrochemical techniques. Among those, linear sweep voltammetry definitely deserves a place even if the principles underlying both methods are fundamentally different.

The characterizing feature of P is the usage, as a working electrode, of

a dropping mercury electrode. This consists of a glass capillary of 3-7
mm external and 0.5 to 0.1 mm internal diameter, connected through a piece
of tubing to a mercury reservoir of varying height, as schematized in Fig. 2.
Drops are continously generated off the lower tip of the capillary, they
grow and eventually fall into the solution under examination. The lifetime
of a single drop depends on a number of factors, such as the height of the
mercury reservoir, the composition of the solution, the applied potential

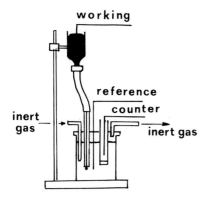

Fig. 2. Polarographic cell.

and so on, and generally varies between 2 and 10 seconds. While applying a
potential difference to the cell such that the dropping electrode takes on,
with respect to the reference electrode, a given potential, the current
flowing in the cell is measured as a function of the dropping electrode
potential. The resultant current-potential curve is called a *polarogram* or
a *polarographic wave*. In Fig. 3 a typical polarogram is shown. A polarogram
(a) is a combination of oscillations, each associated with the growth of
one single drop, with the steep down slope corresponding to the fall of the
drop. Such a polarogram was obtained by applying the increasing potential
slowly and continously, so it is the resultant of the maximum values of many
current-time curves each corresponding to practically constant potential.
The steep rise noticeable in fig. 3 near the end of the potential range covered
is known as *base solution discharge* and sets a natural limit to the accessible
potentials. The potentials range that can be explored is limited by the

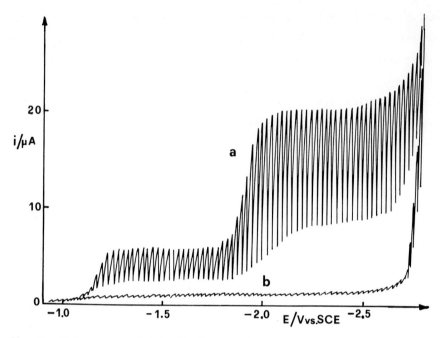

Fig. 3 - Polarograms of (a) nitrobenzene in dimethylformamide solution of 0.1 M Et_4NClO_4; and (b) 0.1 M Et_4NClO_4 in dimethylformamide.

negative part of reduction either of the solvent or of the supporting electrolyte. The latter is an electrolyte added to polarographic system in great excess with respect to electroactive substances. Its function is both to increase the solution conductivity, and to suppress to a negligible level, the mass transport of electroactive substances associated with the electrically induced migration. In a protic solvent the limiting reaction is generally hydrogen evolution. Therefore, in order for an electrode to be of any use in the negative potential region it has to display a considerable overvoltage for hydrogen discharge. Such overvoltage is very low on platinum electrodes but considerably high on mercury. This characteristic, combined with the renewal and reproducibility of dropping electrodes, has tremendously increased the scope of polarography since a rather large window of negative (versus NHE) potentials is thereby accessible and a number of reduction processes have been amenable to analysis. When the solution base discharge limit is reached the current grows exponentially in agreement with the equations previously outlined for the description of electron transfer. On the positive side, similarly, the potential range is limited by the oxidation of the solvent of the supporting electrolyte, or of the very electrode material.

Voltammetric curves

Reversible case. For this kind of process, when the only step contributing to the electrode process beside electron transfer is the mass transport by diffusion and when only the oxidized form is present in solution, the following expression holds for the polarographic wave:

$$E = E_{1/2} - \frac{RT}{nF} \ln \frac{i}{i_d - i} \tag{11}$$

and at 25°C

$$E = E_{1/2} - (0.059/n)\log \frac{i}{i_d - i} \quad V \tag{12}$$

where i_d and $E_{1/2}$ represent respectively the limiting current and the half wave potential, i.e. the potential corresponding to $i_d/2$. If, instantaneous values of current are considered, the following expression holds:

$$i_d = 708nD_0^{1/2} \; C_0^* \; m^{2/3} \; t^{1/6} \tag{13}$$

where n is the number of electrons exchanged, m the rate of flow of mercury (mg/s), D_0 the diffusion coefficient of the substance 0 (cm^2/s) t the drop time (s) and C_0^* the bulk concentration of 0 (millimoles/liter). Relation (13) is called the *Ilkovič equation* after the worker who first solved the diffusion equation. The expression for the half wave potential is:

$$E_{1/2} = E_c^° - \frac{RT}{nF} \ln (D_0/D_R)^{1/2} \tag{14}$$

or at 25°C

$$E_{1/2} = E_c^° - \frac{0.059}{n} \log (D_0/D_R)^{1/2} \quad V \tag{15}$$

where D_0 and D_R are the diffusion coefficients of 0 and R expressed in cm^2/s.

The $E_{1/2}$ is interesting for various reasons. Since it is independent of the characteristics of the capillary and of $C_0^{\ast}$, it is, for a given combination of solvent, supporting electrolyte and temperature, a characteristic of a particular substance. It represents therefore a fingerprint for the identification of the substance. It might be added that the quantity within brackets in (14) and (15) is not very different from unity, leading therefore to the near identification of $E_{1/2}$ with E_c°. Polarographic experiments can consequently often supply this fundamental thermodynamic quantity for a process.

For a reversible process, in particular, one sees from (12) that the plot $E/\log\left[\,i/(i_d-i)\,\right]$ must give a straight line with a slope of 0.059/n V. Finally, considering Eq. 13 one sees i_d to be linearly dependent on the bulk concentration of electroactive substance. This forms the basis for a quantitative analysis application of the technique.

Totally irreversible processes. Consider the reduction of a substance O to another substance R in an electrode processes involving n electrons the only step, other than electron transfer, being mass transport by diffusion. The process is said to be totally irreversible if the effect of the backward electron transfer process can be neglected. In this case the voltammetric curve at 25°C is found to obey Eq. (16):

$$E = E_{1/2} - \frac{0.054}{\alpha n_{\alpha}} \log \frac{i}{i_d - i} \tag{16}$$

$$E_{1/2} = \frac{0.059}{\alpha n_{\alpha}} \log 1.35 \frac{k_{f,h}^{\circ} \cdot t^{1/2}}{D_0^{1/2}} \tag{17}$$

where the symbols have the same meaning as in the reversible case, and n_{α} is the number of electrons involved in the rate determining step. Of course $n_{\alpha} = n$ if the overall electrode reaction occurs, as it has so far been assumed, in a single step. The shape of the wave is similar to the one for reversible processes. Therefore a careful examination is in order before a plot $E/\log \frac{i}{i_d - i}$ can throw light on the nature of a given electrode process. In the totally irreversible case Eq. (17) shows that, in contrast with the behaviour of reversible systems, $E_{1/2}$ is related to electrochemical kinetic parameters and depends on the drop time t. In particular it shifts to more positive values with increasing t. This is to be expected since with increasing t more time is available for the process to reach equilibrium and the potential shifts towards the reversible value. The totally irreversible behaviour is observed in polarography when $k_{s,h} \overset{\sim}{<} 3.10^{-5}$ cm/s.

Application to the study of electrode processes

The first experiment that is generally performed to elucidate an electrode process is the recording of a polarogram, from which much useful information can be obtained. First the number of waves indicates immediately the number of discrete electronic processes taking place in the system. Second, as seen above, the heights and shapes of the waves are related to the number of electrons involved in the overall process and in the rate determining step for any single wave. In particular the existence and the behaviour of the limiting current is highly informative for the identification of the rate determining step. Diagnostic criteria for *diffusion control* are derived from the Ilkovič equation. For example, as a consequence of this equation, one of the tests commonly used consists in determining the limiting current dependence on mercury reservoir height, on which m and t in Eq. (13) depend. For the case of diffusion control the theory predicts a linear i_1 versus $h^{1/2}$ relationship. Also, a temperature increase factor of circa 2%/degree is predicted in the range 20-50°C, as well as a linear $C_0^{::}$ dependence. Deviations from diffusion control of i_1 are generally due to *kinetic processes* or to *adsorption processes*. Generally one refers to *kinetic current* as the current that is obtained in an electrochemical process when the concentration and the concentration gradient of the oxidized or reduced species at the electrode depend not only on the rates of mass transport and of electron transfer but also on the rates of one or a few chemical reactions involving such species and taking place very near the electrode. In general we can write:

$$A \underset{k_2}{\overset{k_1}{\rightleftarrows}} O + ne \underset{k_{b,h}}{\overset{k_{f,h}}{\rightleftarrows}} R \underset{k_4}{\overset{k_3}{\rightleftarrows}} B$$

where the general scheme is liable to very many specializations. Three general
classes can be distinguished, depending on whether the chemical reactions
occur *before, after* or *simultaneously* with the electron transfer. The relative
field is much too vast to explore in a brief presentation (see P references).
It can be said that from the analysis of wave shape and wave height as a
function of various parameters it is often possible to detect the type of
kinetic current at hand. It appears to be reasonable, for instance, that
in general a reaction preceding electron transfer should strongly affect the
value of the limiting current. A slow preceding chemical reaction generally
depressed the limiting current relative to the value it would have had if no
reaction control were there. Also, since chemical rate constants are generally
strongly temperature dependent, the temperature dependence is more pronounced
in the case of chemical rate control. Finally, a dependence of i_l on t is
encountered different from that in the case of diffusion control.

A particularly interesting type of current in case of parallel reaction
control is the one commonly called *catalytic current*. Such currents originate
when the product of electron transfer is converted back to the starting
product through reaction with a reagent present in solution and electroinactive
at the potential explored. This process can be so schematized:

$$O + ne \rightleftarrows R$$
$$\underset{R+Z \xrightarrow{k} O + X}{\qquad}$$

Notice that the overall result is the reduction of Z to X via the redox
system $O + ne \rightleftarrows R$. Henceforth the name of "catalytic process". Since
substance O is regenerated at the electrode it is clear that catalytic current
can be much higher than the one corresponding to k=0. This is the reason
why this behaviour is exploited in analysis with the aim of magnifying
currents due to scarcely concentrated substances which would be undetectable
when controlled by diffusion.

Beside chemical reactions,*adsorption phenomena* can also be extremely
effective versus electrode reactions. These phenomena can be diversified

and complex and no matter how much work has been devoted to them, quite a few problems still await clarification. Essentially two situations are distinguishable whereby polarographic currents may be influenced by absorption. The first relates to the case in which the electroactive substance or its electron reaction product, is the adsorbant, the second to adsorption of other solution components. The first kind of adsorption brings about a separate wave, the so-called adsorption wave. In the second the presence of the adsorbant gives rise to a shifting, deforming or splitting of the wave of the electroactive substance. For example, the splitting of the 4-electron wave normally observed for nitrocompounds in aqueous media, into one 1-electron wave and one 3-electron wave as brought about by surface active agents such as comphor, tylose or gelatine, has been interpreted in terms of inhibition of the radical anion protonation on the electrode surface.

Influence of pH

Among the variable affecting $E_{1/2}$ and i the pH of the system certainly plays a major role. This is related to the possible participation of hydrogen ions in the rate determining step of the redox reaction and with the eventual presence of acid-base equilibria. The pH dependence of $E_{1/2}$ is often utilized to obtain information on the hydrogen ion participation in the electrode reaction. For many reversible and irreversible organic electrode processes of the type

$$0 + ne + pH^+ \rightleftharpoons R$$

the pH dependence of $E_{1/2}$ is given by the relation:

$$\frac{dE_{1/2}}{dpH} = -0.059 \frac{p}{\alpha n_\alpha}$$

where αn_α is replaced by n in the case of reversible processes. A shift of 59 mV per pH unit change is often interpreted to mean that the same number of electrons (n) and of protons (p) are involved in the electrode reaction. When $E_{1/2}$ shifts with pH, the pH of the medium ought to be well controlled in order to prevent local changes in hydrogen ion concentration at mercury drops.

LINEAR SWEEP VOLTAMMETRY

Linear sweep voltammetry (LSV) is an electrochemical relaxation technique. in which the controlled quantity is the potential of a constant surface microelectrode, and the monitored quantity is current versus time. Since the potential varies linearly with time, (see Fig. 4a) the recorded curves

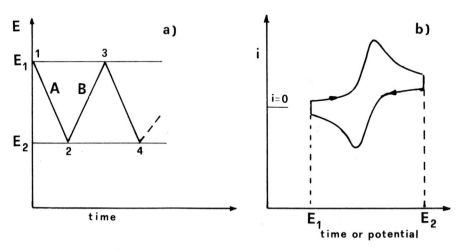

Fig. 4 - Linear sweep voltammetry. a) typical potential wave form used; b) typical variation of current as a function of time or potential.

may also be interpreted as current-potential curves under linearly variable potential (see Fig. 4b). The working electrode potential can be swept in the direction of more negative values (from E_1 to E_2) so that the cathodic branch is observed or in the direction of more positive values (from E_2 to E_1) so that anodic branch is observed. If only one branch of the curve is followed, the A or the B one, the technique is named *single sweep voltammetry* and only the cathodic or the anodic portion of the curve, schematized in Fig. 4b, is observed. If in contrast the potential scanning covers the region 1-3 going through 2, or the region 2-4 going through 3 the name of *cyclic voltammetry* (CV) applies. Generally the waveshape of the potential versus time plot is symmetrical as shown in Fig. 4a. However non symmetrical wave forms, such as slow forward sweep followed by a fast reverse one, can be used to advantage. Since high sweep rates are often used, a cathode ray oscilloscope

is typically used for recording. Cyclic voltammetry represents a more powerful
tool than polarography for the study of electrode processes. In this case
it is possible to vary the potential sweep rate v within a wide range, from
a few mV/s to some thousand V/s. The possibility of reversing, at a stationary
electrode, the sweep direction, allows more detailed information on the
mechanisms of electrode processes to be obtained. For these feature the above
technique is versatile.

Voltammetric curves

 Reversible case. Equations reported below and Fig. 5 describes the wave
shape for a reversible case where the only step, other than electron transfer,
belonging to the overall electrode process, is mass transport through linear,
semiinfinite diffusion, and when only species O is present in solution:

$$i_{pc} = 0.446 \, nFAC_O^* D_O^{1/2} \left(\frac{nFv}{RT}\right)^{1/2}$$

$$E_{pc} = E_{1/2} - 1.11 \frac{RT}{nF}; \quad E_{pa} = E_{1/2} + 1.11 \frac{RT}{nF}; \quad E_{pa} - E_{pc} = 2.22 \frac{RT}{nF}; \quad E_{pc/2} = E_{pa}$$

and at 25°C:

$$i_{pc} = 0.269 \, An^{3/2} C_O^* D_O^{1/2} v^{1/2}$$

$$E_{pc} = E_{1/2} - \frac{0.028}{n} \, V; \quad E_{pa} = E_{1/2} + \frac{0.028}{n} \, V; \quad E_{pa} - E_{pc} = E_{pc/2} - E_{pc} = \frac{0.057}{n} \, V$$

In the above, in addition to symbols already met, one finds the cathodic peak
current i_{pc}, the cathodic half peak current $i_{pc/2}$, the cathodic E_{pc} and the
anodic E_{pa} peak potentials, the cathodic half peak potential $E_{pc/2}$ and the
potential sweep rate v.i$_{pc}$ is in amperes when A, C_O^*, D_O and v are in cm^2, m
mole/l, cm^2/s, and V/s respectively. Recording of the CV curve constitutes
a very good reversibility test. From the above equations it is evident that
for a reversible process the following applies:
a) the cathodic peak has a corresponding anodic peak, with potential circa
   56 mV more positive than the first one;

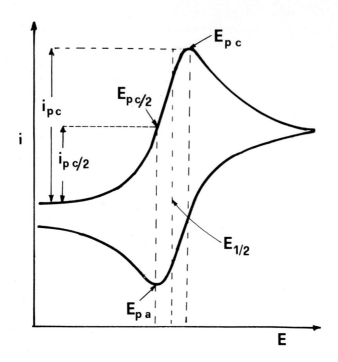

Fig. 5 - Cyclic voltammogram for a reversible process.

b) peak potentials are independent of v;

c) the ratio $i_{pc}/v^{1/2}$ is independent of v.

The expression $i_{pc}/v^{1/2}$ is often called the current function, and its dependence on v is a source of detailed information on the electrode process. Furthermore it can be shown that the reverse peak current i_{pa} and the forward peak current i_{pc} are equal when measured from the extension of the forward curve. Finally, the valence of the electrode process n and the half wave potential $E_{1/2}$, henceforth E_c°, can be deduced. The kinetic parameters on the other hand cannot.

Totally irreversible case. In the totally irreversible reduction case a major characteristic is the lack of any anodic peak on the reverse sweep and similarly for an irreversible oxidation, the lack of any reduction step on the forward sweep. Concerning the observed reduction (oxidation) peak, its waveshape is characterized:

$$i_{pc} = 0.496nFAC_0^* D_0^{1/2} \left(\frac{\alpha n_\alpha Fv}{RT}\right)^{1/2}$$

$$E_{pc} = E_c^\circ - \frac{RT}{\alpha n_\alpha F} \left[0.78 + \ln \left(\frac{\alpha n_\alpha Fv}{RT}\right)^{1/2} - \ln \frac{k_{s,h}}{D_0^{1,2}} \right]$$

where the symbols above have the same meaning as previously given. These
equations show that, as in the reversible case, the current function $i_p/v^{1/2}$
is independent of v. In contrast, E_{pc} becomes more negative with increasing
v. These equations show that in this case it is possible to obtain kinetic
parameters αn_α and $k_{s,h}$ which characterize the electron transfer process.

Other types of electrode processes. Another type of behaviour which is
frequently encountered and which contributes to the potential of the technique
is illustrated in Fig. 6. As is shown, while at low sweep rates no oxidation
peak is observed on the anodic branch, with increasing v an oxidation peak is
observed so that eventually a diffusion controlled reversible process type
of curve is obtained. Such a pattern is normally associated with an electrode
process in which a chemical reaction follows the electron transfer: (process
EC, where E stands for electrochemical, C for chemical step).

$$0 + ne \rightleftharpoons R \qquad \text{(E step)}$$

$$R \xrightarrow{k} \text{products (C step)}$$

The v dependence of the curves observed can be easily explained in terms of
this mechanism. At low v's, R is not available for oxidation since the

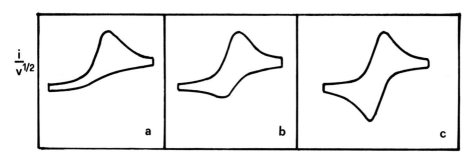

Fig. 6 - Cyclic voltammetric curves for an EC process. The scan rate increases
from a) to c).

chemical reaction is fast enough to consume it in the course of the sweep. Viceversa, for high v's, very little reaction takes place and R can be reoxidized so that the reversible pattern appears. The study of this behaviour as a function of v often allows the determination of the rate constant of the coupled chemical reaction. If one compares the totally irreversible case due to slow electron transfer with the case in which irreversibility is caused by a subsequent chemical reaction one can usually discriminate between them on the ground of the v dependence. In the first case the anodic peak will always be absent whereas in the second, it may or may not appear depending on the values of v and k. Many other mechanisms have been examined in the last few years. Due to space limitations the reader is referred to the abundant literature on the subject (LSV references).

CONTROLLED POTENTIAL ELECTROLYSIS AND COULOMETRY

It must emphasised that whenever an electrode mechanism is proposed it should be supported with experimental evidence such as the identification of the products of the mechanism. In this context the use of *controlled potential electrolysis* (CPE) for producing large enough quantities of products to be amenable to usual chemical and spectroscopic analysis is useful.

Of course caution must be exercised in establishing correlations between micro and macro phenomena. Although the same electrode process is usually observed in both kinds of experiments, factors such as electrolysis time, electrode surface, concentration, pH, can cause relevant differences between the two types of phenomena. For example many chemical reactions that in voltammetric experiments are too slow to occur show up in CPE, in view of the much longer time scale and thus give rise to very different results. Furthermore it might be pointed out that CPE, beside being a very useful technique for the study of electrode processes, is also unique for the degree of selectivity it offers in the realization of specific oxidations or reductions, a selectivity certainly unequalled by chemical reagents.

Finally a word should be said about *coulometry* i.e. the determination of the total charge exchanged during electrolysis. This, together with the

recording of electrolysis current versus time, can yield important information
on electrode processes. In fact the charge exchanged can be related to n, the
number of electrons exchanged per mole of electroactive substance. Results
can be compared with the quantities determined by means of P and CV. If
the micro and macro experiments results do not coincide, this is a strong
indication that secondary chemical processes, competing pathways etc. are
involved.

UTILIZATION OF THE TECHNIQUES PREVIOUSLY DESCRIBED IN THE STUDY OF PROBELMS
INVOLVED WITH CHEMICAL RADIOSENSITIZATION OF HYPOXIC CELLS
Correlation of voltammetric results with pulse radiolysis data of nitrocompounds
and radiosensitizers[1]

   There is good evidence that some physico-chemical properties of
nitrocompounds, and in particular of nitroimidaoles, such as one-electron
reduction potentials, can be correlated with the efficiences of these compounds
as hypoxic cell radiosensitizers. One electron reduction potentials of various
sensitizers have been measured in aqueous solution utilizing pulse radiolysis
techniques. In this connection, the usual electrochemical techniques may be
less useful because of the limited stability in aqueous media of the radical
produced by electron transfer from the electrode. The first one-electron step
is often not detectable and the reduction appears to be irreversible.
Furthermore in such media adsorption phenomena often occur which interfere with
the electrode process.

   In formally aprotic media, however, the radicals formed may be sufficiently
stable and since absorption does not play an important role, one-electron
reversible steps may be readily observed. For these reasons, we have studied
the reduction of a series of nitro-compounds by cyclic voltammetry in dimethylformamide (DMF). The purpose of this investigation was to establish whether a
correlation exist between the redox data obtained with our method and the
redox data obtained by pulse radiolysis.

   The list of the compounds studied is reported in Tab. 3 of Prof. Breccia's
lecture in this Volume.

The seven nitrocompounds identified in the list by the symbols B,Q,E, Ro-0482, DA 3837, DA 3829 and Flagyl, all of which had been previously investigated by pulse radiolysis technique, the first five by Wardman et al.[2] and the last two by Breccia et al.[3] show a first one-electron reversible reduction process in the range of the potential sweep rate v explored: 0.1 - - 60V/s. The nature of the process has been established on the basis of the usual criteria (see eq.s under reversible case in LSV).

For the one-electron reversible reduction of the compound S to a species S^-, in the absence of complications due to adsorption processes, the $E_{p,c}$ can be expressed[4] as

$$E_{p,c} = E° -1,11(RT/F) + (RT/F)\ln(f_S D_S^{-1/2}/f_{S^-}D_S^{-1/2}) \qquad (18)$$

$$FE° = A_S - \delta_{S^-}° - C° \qquad (19)$$

where E° is the standard potential***, A_S the electron affinity of S, δ_{S^-} the differential real free energy of solvation of the ion S^- of the species S, D's and f's the respective diffusion and activity coefficients; C° is a constant appropriate to the reference electrode employed and which includes liquid junction potentials; R, T and F have the usual significance. Implicit in the above equations is the assumption that additional terms relative to the free energy of complex formation with the solvent or supporting electrolyte or between radical ions and their counter-ions can be neglected. Obviously, the variation of the solvent can change all the values in the above equations except that of A_S. In this regard, on the basis of Eq. (18) and (19), the cathodic peak potential determined in DMF, $E_{p,c}^{DMF}$, will be related to the one determined in water $E_{p,c}^W$ through the relation:

$$E_{p,c}^{DMF} = E_{p,c}^W + \Delta\delta_{S^-} + \Delta C + (RT/F)\Delta\ln(f,D) \qquad (20)$$

where $\Delta\delta_{S^-} = \delta_{S^-}°(w) - \delta_S°(DMF)$

$$\Delta C = C°(w) - C°(DMF)$$

*** The superscript o is used to denote a standard state.

$$\Delta \ln(f,D) = \ln(f_S D_S^{-1/2} / f_S - D_S^{1/2})_{DMF} - \ln(f_S D_S^{-1/2} / f_S - D_S^{1/2})_W$$

If it is assumed that the Δ terms in Eq. (20) are reasonable constant for all compounds in the series, the $E_{p,c}^{DMF}$ will differ from $E_{p,c}^{W}$ by a constant quantity for the various compounds and a linear correlation between $E_{p,c}^{DMF}$ and the one electron reduction potential E_7^1 determined in water by pulse radiolysis should be expected.

In Fig. 7 by full circoles the peak potentials $E_{p,c}^1$ for the first cathodic process of the compounds showing a first reversible reduction process in DMF are plotted against the one electron reduction potentials E_7^1 as determined by pulse radiolysis (full circles). As can be seen these points can

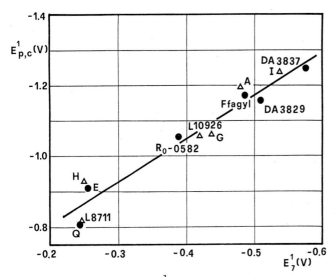

Fig. 7 - Peak potentials $E_{p,c}^1$ for the first cathodic process, measured in this work, reported against one-electron potentials E_7^1 from pulse radiolysis; ($\bullet$) reversible, (Δ) not reversible.

satisfactorly fit a straight line, with a correlation coefficient of 0.98. Although the number of compounds investigated is limited, the goodness of fit supports the hypothesis that voltammetric reduction potentials might be utilized to get information on the efficiency of the relevant compound as a radiosensitizer, and provide an alternative to the use of pulse radiolysis data.

In Fig. 7 the peak potential values for the other compounds of the list are shown triangles. The first reduction peaks of these compounds are irreversible up to the maximum utilized scan rate (60,V/s). Clearly these points do not deviate appreciably from the straight line previously obtained on the basis of reversible potential data. Apparently the degree of irreversibility does not bring about a change from reversible potentials such as to cause a significant variation of the correlation coefficient in the specific case . Other electrochemical investigations are, however, necessary to clarify the nature of the irreversibility observed and thus to assess the meaning of the observed $E_{p,c}^1$.

Electrochemical study of the interaction between cells and radiosensitizers[5]

Various mechanisms have been proposed to explain the radiosensitization due to electron affinic radiosensitizers. Fundamentally they are: (1) capture of electrons of the cellular target molecule by the radiosensitizer to prevent charge neutralization processes within the target molecule; (2) radical fixation through addition reactions of radiosensitizer molecules with radicals produced on target biomolecules; (3) formation of stable cytoxic products; (4) attack on biomolecules from transient radicals of the sensitizer.

While all proposed mechanisms are likely to come into play and produce the overall effect of radiosensitization upon irradiation treatment, most data in the literature support the first two as being the major mechanisms in the process. Recently, however, by utilizing UV light, which is much more specific in its action than ionizing radiation, it has been shown[6] that the fourth mechanism can contribute as well to the lethal effect of radiosensitizing agents on cells through the action of short lived excited states or free radicals species of sensitizer with biological molecules and other radicals also formed.

In relation to the elucidation of such processes and of the role that

the species produced by the radiosensitizer can play in cellular radiosensitization, electrochemical techniques can be helpful. Essentially
this study can be done in two ways, either by examining the modification of
voltammetric curves of the radiosensitizers after addition of cells, or by
generating at an electrode, the reduction products of the radiosensitizer
and studying their interactions with the cells or with model biological
systems. It might be noted that this kind of study could also help in
clarifying the mechanism of any interaction between membranes and sensitizers.

In the following the preliminary results of an electrochemical study of
the interaction between selected nitroimidazoles and Euglena gracilis Z.
cells, carried out by using controlled potential electrolysis and coulometry
are described. The cell was chosen first because it had been utilized in
other investigations and also because of some favourable properties such ease of
reproduction, simplicity of culture medium, good resistance to the modifying
effects of variables, such as pH. As a working electrode, a mercury electrode
was chosen in view of its properties previously described in the polarography
section. Survival tests of cells in the presence of Hg were carried out by
allowing them to sit on a Hg pool for a three times as long as the electrolysis
time. No effect on their growth was detected.

The following solutions, buffered with 0.1 M phosphate buffer to a pH=7.2
and deaerated with N_2, were electrolized at a controlled potential of
-0.650 V vs. SCE, corresponding to the current plateau observed after a
pronounced maximum for the reduction of Flagyl (1(ethyl-β-hydroxyl)-2-methyl-
5-nitroimidazole): (a) buffer solution; (b) buffer solution + cells; (c) buffer
solution + Flagyl (1.10^{-3}M); (d) buffer solution + Flagyl (1.10^{-3}M) + cells.
Results show firstly, that the charge exchanged upon electrolyzing for the
same time solutions (a) and (b) for a similar period is the same. This
indicates that the cells are not electroactive at those potentials in agreement
with the polarogram recorded for solution (b). Secondly, it is observed
that after flow of equal quantities of charge (1 coulomb) by controlled
potential electrolysis on solutions (c) and (b), the Flagyl concentration
present at the end of the experiment with solution (d) is higher than the
corresponding quantity in case (c). In particular, the apparent number

of electrons exchanged per molecule of Flagyl n_{app} is 2.9 for solution (c) and 4.2. for solution (d). These results show clearly that there is interaction between the reduction products of Flagyl and the cells.

In order to investigate the nature of interaction, survival test of the cells were carried out. In particular the comparison between survival tests of cells contained in the electrolyzed solutions (d) and (b) show that the survival is much lower for solution (d) than for solution (b). Since Flagyl and its final electrolysis products have no appreciable lethal effect upon the cells, the results show that this effect is due to one or more reduction intermediates of Flagyl.

Analogous results have been obtained with L8711 (1-metyl-5-formyl-2nitro-imidazole). In particular, the value of n_{app} obtained from solution containing in addition to the base electrolyte, L8711 and the cells, is also higher (for comparable amounts of charge flow) than the one obtained from the solution containing L8711 and no cells. Likewise, the survival of cells in the solution containing L8711 electrolyzed at constant potential, appears to be much lower than solutions not containing L8711.

The results indicate that the fourth mechanism may contribute to the lethal effects of radiosensitizer.

Further experiments are in progress aiming at the identification of the species responsible for lethal action.

REFERENCES

1. Breccia, A., Roffia, S. and Berilli, S., Int. J. Radiat. Biol., in press.
2. Wardman, P. and Clarke, E.D., J. Chem. Faraday Trans., I, 72, 1377 (1976).
3. Breccia, A. and Busi, F., work in progress.
4. Case, B., Hush, N.S., Parsons, R. and Peover, M.E., J. Electroanal. Chem., 10, 360 (1965).
5. Roffia, S., Gattavecchia, E. and Breccia, A., work in progress.
6. Fischer, G.J., Watts, M.E., Patel, K.B. and Adams, G.E., Br. J. Cancer, 37, (III) 111 (1978).

Electrochemical theory

Delahay, P., New Instrumental Methods in Electrochemistry, Interscience
New York, 1954.

Delahay, P., Double layer and Electrode Kinetics, Interscience, New York,
1965.

Vetter, K.G., Electrochemical Kinetics, Academic Press, New York, 1967.

Koryta, J., Dvorak, J. and Bohackova, V., Electrochemistry, Methuen and
Co., London, 1970.

Bockris, J.O.M. and Reddy, A.K.N., Modern Electrochemistry, Plenum Press,
New York, 1972.

Bianchi, G. and Mussini, T., Elettrochimica, Tamburini-Masson ed., Milan,
1976.

Polarography

Kolthoff, I.M. and Lingane, J.J., Polarography, 2nd ed., Interscience, New
York, 1952.

Meites, L., Polarographic Techniques, 2nd ed., Interscience, New York, 1965.

Heyrovsky, J. and Kuta, J., Principles of Polarography, Academic Press,
New York, 1966.

Linear sweep voltammetry

Matsuda, H. and Ayabe, Y., Z. Electrochem., 59, 494 (1955).

Nicholson, R.S. and Shain, I., Anal. Chem., 36, 706 (1964).

Savéant, J.M. and E. Vianello, Electrochim. Acta, 8, 905 (1963); 12, 1545
(1967); 10, 905 (1965).

Wopschall, R.H. and Shain, I., Anal. Chem., 39, 1514 (1967).

Mastragostino, M., Nadjo, L. and Savéant, J.M., Electrochim. Acta, 13, 721
(1968).

Nadjo, L. and Savéant, J.M., J. Electroanal. Chem., 44, 327 (1973).

Andrieux, C.P. and Savéant, J.M. Electroanal. Chem., 53, 165 (1974).

Potential controlled electrolysis and coulometry

Bard, A.J. and Santhanam, J.S.V., in Electroanal. Chemistry, (Bard, A.J.
ed.) vol. 4, Dekker, New York, 1970, p. 215.

58

Organic and inorganic electrochemistry texbooks some of which contain extensive introductions to the techniques described in the present exposition.

Zuman, P., Elucidation of Organic Electrode Processes, Academic Press, New York, 1968.

Headridge, J.B., Electrochemical Techniques for Inorganic Chemists, Academic Press, New York, 1969.

Mann, C.K. and Barnes, K.K., Electrochemical Reactions in non Aqueous Systems, Dekker, New York, 1970.

Tomilov, A.P., Mairanovskii, S.G., Fioshin, M.Ya. and Smirnov, V.A., The Electrochemistry of Organic Compounds, Halsted Press, New York, 1972.

Organic Electrochemistry, ed. by Baizer, M.M., Dekker, New York, 1973.

Rifi, M.R. and Covitz, F.H., Introduction to Organic Electrochemistry, Dekker, New York, 1974.

PULSE RADIOLYSIS TECHNIQUE

F. BUSI

Laboratorio di Fotochimica e Radiazioni di alta energia, C.N.R., Via
Castagnoli 3, Bologna, Italy.

GENERAL

The chimical or biological changes induced by high energy radiation are
the synthesis of a complex series of processes which follow the primary act
of energy transfer from the radiation to the molecules of the absorbing
material. Energy transfer occurs through excitation and ionization of the
molecules in the vicinity of the radiation trajectory. The primary
excited molecules, ions and ejected electrons are generally highly unstable
and undergo fast secondary reactions which ultimately lead to the final
stable products. The study of the biological response to high energy radiation
includes the identification of the final products and the mechanism of their
formation. The steady state irradiation method is normally used for the
determination of the final products and their yields by conventional
chemical analysis of the system after irradiation. The irradiation time is
generally much longer than the lifetime of the transients and the dose rate
$/$ energy transferred to the irradiated system per unit time $/$ is relatively
low. Therefore, the low steady state concentrations of the transients do
not allow their direct observation. The concentration limit for the
detection of a chemical species by fast physico-chemical methods is 10^{-7} -
- 10^{-6} M. Using a ^{60}Co gamma-cell as a steady state irradiation source,
with a typical dose rate D = 10^{17} e V/cc/s, for a species X with a yield
G = 1 $/$ the G gives the number of particles formed for each 100 eV of
energy absorbed by the system $/$ and a rate constant of second order
disappearance of 10^{10} M^{-1} s^{-1}, the steady state concentration is given by

$$\frac{d \, / \, X \, /}{d \, t} = \frac{D \times G \times 10^3}{100 \times N} \times 10^{10} \, / \, X \, /^2 = 0 \qquad (1)$$

where N is the Avogadro's number, from which it can be shown

$$\underline{/}^-X_\underline{/}^- = 1.3 \times 10^{-8} \text{ M} \tag{2}$$

which is a concentration too low to be detected.

Pulse radiolysis employs an intense pulse of radiation whose duration is normally shorter than the lifetime of the intermediates. A single pulse can produce concentrations of intermediates which are high enough to be studied by fast physico-chemical techniques. A typical value of the dose absorbed by a system irradiated with a 50 ns. pulse of 12 MeV electrons from a linear accelerator is 10^{17} eV/cc which corresponds to a concentration of the intermediate X

$$\underline{/}^-X_\underline{/}^- \quad \frac{\text{Dose} \times \text{G} \times 10^3}{\text{N} \times 100} = 2.5 \times 10^{-6} \text{ M} \tag{3}$$

The lifetime of X is under these conditions

$$t_{\frac{1}{2}} = 1/10^{10} \times 2.5 \times 10^{-6} = 40 \text{ }\mu\text{s} \tag{4}$$

Since the response time of fast optical detection techniques is of the order of nanoseconds, the kinetics of processes with lifetimes of tens of nanoseconds can be observed directly.

The radiation pulse is obtained from an electron accelerator. Several types of electron accelerators are now available. We will briefly describe two types of accelerators: the microwave linear accelerator and the Febetron 705-B. The source of energy used to accelerate the electrons in a linear accelerator, is a klystron oscillator which produces pulses of radiofrequency power. These pulses are supplied to a waveguide in which the acceleration takes place. Electrons from a high current electron gun are injected axially into the microwave field in the waveguide. The waveguide contains a large number of circular irises whose spacing varies along its length. The spacing determines the wave velocity and is designed so that the wave velocity increases as the electrons are accelerated. The electrons which enter at the correct phase, ride in closepacked "bunches" on the wave-fronts of the

electromagnetic waves and are continously in an accelerating field. The
linear accelerators produce either single pulses, whose duration can vary
from 5 ns to 5 μs, or trains of pulses of repetition rates up to ∿ 1000
per second.

The Febetron 705-B electron accelerator is an impulse generator employing
a Marx surge circuit. It basically consists of a stack of eighty condenser
modules and an evacuated field emission tube. The condenser bank is charged
to 20-25 KV in parallel and by means of a 10 KV trigger pulse is discharged
in series. The 1-2 MeV pulse generated is applied to the cathode of the
field emission tube which emits an electron pulse of 30 ns. The maximum
dose obtainable from the Febetron 705-B is ∿ 8 M rads per pulse while the
one from a 50 ns pulse generated in a linear accelerator is ∿ 10 Krads. The
high electron beam current that the Febetron can provide, circa 6000 amps
per 30 ns pulse at 2 MeV, makes possible the use of this machine for X-ray
pulse radiolysis. The X ray dose obtainable is ∿ 1 Krad per 30 ns pulse.
The X ray pulse is generated by bremsstrahlung effect on a tungsten target
attached over the anode of the electron emission tube.

The detection methods most commonly used in pulse radiolysis to investigate
the properties of transient chemical species produced by the radiation pulse
include kinetic spectrophotometry, flash spectroscopy, measurements of
light emission in the spectral range from the ultraviolet to the infrared,
studies of transient electrical conductivity and recently of the polarographic
behaviour of the transients.

KINETIC SPECTROPHOTOMETRY

a) Absorption

The kinetic spectrophotometry detection method is based on the quantitative
measurements of absorption signals, at a fixed wavelength, due to optically
absorbing chemical species produced by the pulse or present in the irradiated
system. The apparatus used to monitor the changes in the absorption signal

is a form of spectrophotometer and is schematically shown in figure 1. The
analysing light traverses a quartz cell fitted with optical windows
perpendicular to the direction of the light beam and contraining the sample.
The wavelength of interest is selected by means of the monochromator. The
selected wavelength is focused on to a detector, photomultiplier or
photodiode. The anode of the photomultiplier is earthed through a resistence,
R, and connected to a cathode ray oscilloscope. The value of the photocurrent
before irradiation, which is recorded on a voltmeter, is the reference and
only changes in transmission with respect to this reference are recorded on
the oscilloscope. The response time of the system depends on the characteristics
of the photomultiplier and on the value of the resistence, R, and it can be
as fast as a few nanoseconds.

As an example of the application of this method let us consider the
irradiation of an aqueous solution of the ionic specie A^+. The radiolysis of
water can be schematically represented by reaction 1-9:

(1) $\quad H_2O \quad \xrightarrow{\text{radiation}} \quad H_2O^+ + e^-$

(2) $\quad\qquad\qquad \longrightarrow \quad H_2O\colon\colon$

(3) $\quad H_2O^+ + H_2O \quad \longrightarrow \quad H_3O^+ + OH$

(4) $\quad H_2O\colon\colon \quad \longrightarrow \quad H + OH$ (or $H_2 + O$ negligible)

(5) $\quad e^- + n\ H_2O \quad \longrightarrow \quad e^-_{aq}$ (hydrated electron)

(6) $\quad H_3O^+ + e^-_{aq} \quad \longrightarrow \quad H + H_2O$

(7) $\quad OH + H \quad \longrightarrow \quad H_2O$

(8) $\quad OH + OH \quad \longrightarrow \quad H_2O_2$

(9) $\quad H + H \quad \longrightarrow \quad H_2$

Suppose that the solute A^+ undergose a fast reaction with the hydrated
electron

(10) $\qquad A^+ + e^-_{aq} \quad \longrightarrow \quad A$

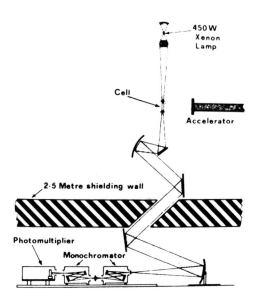

450 W
Xenon
Lamp

Cell

Accelerator

2·5 Metre shielding wall

Photomultiplier

Monochromator

Fig. 1. Schematic layout of optical system.

The presence of A^+ increases the rate of disappearance of e^-_{aq}. The decay of the hydrated electron is given by

$$- \frac{d \, [e^-_{aq-}]}{dt} = k_{10} \, [A^+] \, [e^-_{aq-}] + k_6 \, [e^-_{aq-}] \, [H_3O^+] \qquad (5)$$

For the doses normally used, as a first approximation, for neutral solutions, $[e^-_{aq-}] = [H_3O^+]$.

If $[A^+] \gg [e^-_{aq-}]$ the concentration of the solute A^+ may be assumed constant and equation 6 becomes

$$- \frac{d \, [e^-_{aq-}]}{dt} = k \, [e^-_{aq-}] + k_6 \, [e^-_{aq-}]^2 \qquad (6)$$

here $k = k_{10} \, [A^+]$. The second term in the right hand side is negligible compared to the first since $[e^-_{aq-}]$ is small, therefore the differential rate equations is

$$- \frac{d \left[e_{aq-} \right]}{dt} = k \left[e_{aq-} \right] \tag{7}$$

Integration of eq. 7 gives

$$\ln \left[e_{aq-} \right]_t - \ln \left[e_{aq-} \right]_o = - kt \tag{8}$$

where $\left[e_{aq-} \right]_t$ and $\left[e_{aq-} \right]_o$ are the concentrations at time t and at time zero respectively.

The hydrated electron presents a characteristic absorption spectrum in the visible with a peak at 7200 $\overset{o}{A}$, figure 2. Therefore the kinetics of the decay of the hydrated electron can be followed by kinetic spectrophotometry. If at the selected wavelength e_{aq}^- absorbs and A^+ and A do not, $\left[e_{aq-} \right]$ can be expressed in terms of the optical density OD, from Beer's law:

$$OD = \ln \frac{I_o}{I} = \varepsilon \left[e_{aq-} \right] 1 \tag{9}$$

where I_o and I are the intensities of the transmitted light in the absence or presence of e_{aq}^- at a concentration $\left[e_{aq-} \right]$, ε is the optical extintion coefficient of e_{aq}^- and 1 is the optical path length. Equation 9 can be written

$$\ln OD_t - \ln OD_o = - kt \tag{10}$$

A plot of $\ln OD_t$ vs t gives straight line and the slope gives the rate constant k. If at the selected wavelength, e_{aq}^- and A^+ do not absorb and A absorbs and is a stable product, the integrated equation is

$$\ln (OD_\infty - OD_t) - \ln OD = - kt \tag{11}$$

where OD_∞ represents the optical density of the solution when reaction 10 is complete. A plot of $\ln (OD_\infty - OD_t)$ vs t gives a straight line and the slope gives the rate constant k. Equations 11 and 12 apply to first order and pseudo-first order processes.

Suppose that the product A, or any other radiolysisi product, is unstable and decays by reaction 11

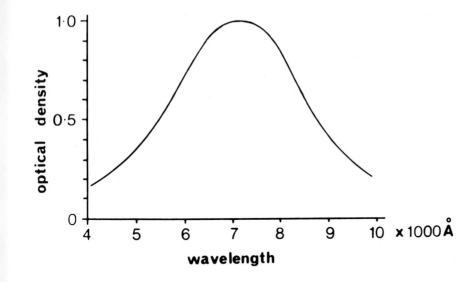

Fig. 2. Absorption spectrum of the hydrated electron

$$(11) \qquad\qquad 2\ A \longrightarrow P$$

The rate equation for disapperance of A is

$$- \frac{d\ \underline{/}\ \bar{A}\ \underline{/}}{dt} = 2\ k_{11}\ \underline{/}\ \bar{A}\ \underline{/}^{\ 2} \qquad\qquad (12)$$

Integration of equation 12 gives

$$\frac{1}{\underline{/}\ \bar{A}\ \underline{/}} - \frac{1}{\underline{/}\ \bar{A}\ \underline{/}_o} = 2\ k_{11}\ t \qquad\qquad (13)$$

If at the selected wavelength A absorbs and P does not, equation 14 may be written

$$\frac{1}{OD_t} - \frac{1}{OD_o} = (\frac{2\ k_{11}}{A_1})\ t \qquad\qquad (14)$$

If P absorbs and A does not

$$\frac{1}{(OD_\infty - OD_t)} - \frac{1}{OD} = (\frac{4\ k_{11}}{P_1})\ t \qquad\qquad (15)$$

Equations 14 and 15 apply to second order reactions. The absolute rate constant may be calculated from the slope of the plot $\dfrac{1}{OD_t}$ vs t or $\dfrac{1}{(OD_\infty - OD_t)}$ vs t only if the absorption coefficient or the concentration of the observed species at some specific time is known.

The optical spectrum of a transient can be obtained by recording the variation of the absorption signal with time at different wavelengths and plotting the OD_t a fixed time for the different wavelengths.

b) Emission

An appreciable fraction of the energy transferred to the irradiated system from the incident radiation may result in direct excitation of the molecules. In addition, excited molecules may be formed by secondary processes such as ion recombination or energy transfer from one component of the system to another. Excited molecules are unstable and dissipate the excess energy by photochemical processes, by energy transfer processes, or through radiative or radiationless transition to the ground state. Measurement of emitted light is the most sensitive optical detection method even if the fraction of excited molecules that dissipate the excess energy by emission of light is generally low. The probability that one excited molecule will emit light is independent of the presence of the other excited molecules. In other words luminescence is a first order process. Therefore the intensity of the light emitted at any time is proportional to the number, N_t, of excited molecules present at that time:

$$- \frac{dN}{dt} = k_1 N \tag{16}$$

Integration leads to the equation

$$N_t = N_o \, e^{-k_1 t} \tag{17}$$

or

$$I_t = I_o \, e^{-k_1 t} \tag{18}$$

where I_t and I_o are the intensity at the time t and zero respectively.
Equation 18 may be written

$$\ln I_t - \ln I_o = - k_1 t \qquad (19)$$

A plot of $\ln I_t$ vs t gives a straight line of which the slope gives the
first order rate constant for the luminescence.

FLASH SPECTROSCOPY

The menthod is based on the detection of the absorbtion spectrum of any
products formed by irradiation.

The equipment consists of a spectrograph, a short-duration flash light
source giving a broad continous spectrum and suitable trigger and delay
circuits, figure 3. To follow the kinetics of a reaction, spectrograms
may be recorded at different the intervals after the radiation pulse by
changing the delay between the electron pulse and the light flash. The rates
of reaction can be more easily determined by using the kinetic spectrophotometry
technique.

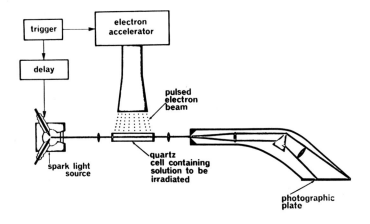

Fig. 3. Pulse radiolysis equipment for spectrographic recording of transient
absorbing species.

CONDUCTIVITY

The ionization produced by the radiation pulse results in a change in
the electrical conductivity of the irradiated system. The measurement of
the radiation-induced conductivity and the mobilities of the ions formed
give valuable information about the behaviour of ions and electrons in the
irradiated system. The interpretation of conductivity data is complicated
by the fact that the observed signal is the sum of the contributions all ions
present in the system. This represents a serious limitation since the
individual species cannot be separately monitored. Figure 4 shows
schematically an experimental apparatus for conductivity measurements.

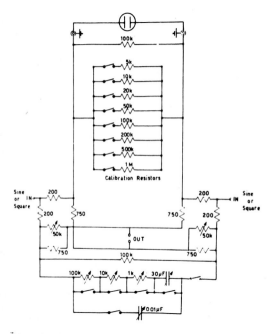

Fig. 4. Conductivity measuring circuit for condumetric pulse radiolysis.

The measuring circuit is essentially a modified Wheatshone bridge. The
voltage applied to the cell may be kept constant for the time of observation,
is the DC method. In the AC method, a periodic voltage, i.e. sine wave, is
applied to the cell with a high frequency with respect to the observation

time. To avoid electrode polarization in aqueous solutions, a suitable
circuit reverses the voltage polarity at a variable frequency.

The molar conductivity, Λ, which represents the conducting power of all
ions produced by 1 mole of electrolyte in a given solution, is given by

$$\Lambda = \frac{F}{10^3} \sum_i \underline{/}\,c_{i-}\underline{/}\, z_i\, u_i \qquad (20)$$

where F is the Faraday, $\underline{/}\,c_{i-}\underline{/}$ the molar concentration of the charged species
i, z_i the charge and u_i the mobility which represents the speed with which
an ion moves under a potential gradient of one volt per cm. The radiation
induces a conductivity change $\Delta\Lambda$, due to the ions formed or to the ions
already present whose concentration changes as a result of reaction with
radiolysis products:

$$\Delta\Lambda = \frac{F}{10^3} \sum_i \underline{/}\,c_{i-}\underline{/}_t\, z_i\, u_i \qquad (21)$$

$\underline{/}\,c_{i-}\underline{/}_t$ is the concentration at time t. If $\Delta\Lambda$ is due to a single ion
pair, and the positive and negative ion are produced with the same yield,
evaluation of the data gives the kinetic and the electrochemical properties
of the ions which are necessary for the study of the irradiated system.

POLAROGRAPHY

The principle of this method consists of the detection of short-lived
intermediates on the basis of their redox behaviour to a mercury drop electrode.
The advantages of this technique are:

a) the investigation of the redox behaviour of short-lived transients;

b) the determination of the rate constant of the electron transfer process;

c) the determination of diffusion coefficients of radicals.

At first, polarography was applied to pulse radiolysis[1] using a "quasi"
potentiostatic technique, figure 5. Rather large doses are delivered to
the sample contained in a three electrode polarographic cell. Current-time
curves are recorded at either a DME or HMDE electrode following the irradiation
of the electrode and adjacent solution.

The results obtained with this method, despite the necessity of using a

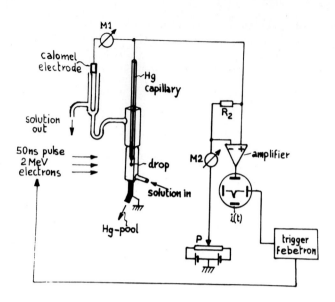

Fig. 5. Pulse radiolysis equipment for polarographic measurements of transient species.

high dose under unsophisticated potentiostatic conditions to obtain an adequately large signal-to-noise ratio, have estabilished unambiguously the important rôle that current measurements can play in the clarification of radiation-induced chemical or biological effects. Recently a new technique has been developed which calls for radiation doses of the order of 300 rads and with a rise time of the order of 5-10 μs. Measurements are made of the change in the voltage between the DME and the unirradiated mercury pool electrode after a pulse X ray delivered at a fixed time in the DME drop-life, under "quasi" coulostatic conditions. The voltage change is amplified by a specially designed low noise solid state amplifier by a factor of 300 before being passed to an oscilloscope. The coulostatic change in interfacial potential, when only one species is involved in the faradaic reaction at the electrode surface, is given by

$$
d E = 1/C_{dl}^{\circ} \int_{o}^{t} n \, FD \left(\frac{\delta \bar{/ C \, /}}{\delta x} \right)_{x=o} dt
\tag{22}
$$

where $\underline{/}C\underline{/}$ is the concencentration of the reactant species, D its diffusion coefficient, n the number of electron involved in the faradaic process, F is the Faraday, and C_{dl}° is the specific differential capacity. If the dose is uniform, if the faradaic process is diffusion-controlled and if there is no loss of any intermediate by reaction in the solution, the signal is proportional to $t^{\frac{1}{2}}$. In this case the slopes of the plots faradaic-charge vs $t^{\frac{1}{2}}$ at potential where the current is diffusion controlled is given by

$$\text{Slope} = K \underline{/} C \underline{/} D^{\frac{1}{2}} \qquad (23)$$

where $K = 1/C_{dl}^{\circ} nF$. By comparing the slope of this plot for a species whose value of D has been determined and K can be calculated, with the slopes for transients whose diffusion coefficients are unknown, these coefficients can be calculated. Unfortunately the simple case of absence of reactions in solution for the reactant at the electrode is the exception rather than the rule. Generally potential change-time data may be analysed quantitatively using a calculator and iterative finite difference programs which take account of linear diffusion of electrochemically active intermediates in the presence of complications introduced by the reaction of intermediates in the solution.

RAPID MIXING TECHNIQUE

The rapid mixing technique has been found to be extremely useful for the study of the mechanisms of the biological response to radiation. The radiation perturbation is followed, or preceded, by the admission into the biological system of some chemical modifying substance. Figure 6 shows the rapid mixing apparatus. A small mixing chamber is connected to two syringes by means of fine capillary tubing. Compression of the two syringes simultaneously drives the liquid contents rapidly into the mixing chamber. Pneumatic techniques are employed to produce a push of half a ton and enable the flow rate to be easely adjusted up to a maximum of 1 cm a ms. The combined solution, after irradiation, is collected in another syringe and is available for assay. The analysis of the radiation-induced biological modification in experiments where the chemical perturbation occurs at different times before and after irradiation gives formation on whether or not the

radiobiological mechanism involves chemical free radical precursors. It
has been found, for example, that oxygen is able to modify the radio-
-sensitivity of bacteria even if is mixed with the solution a few milliseconds
before irradiation. Such results clearly demonstrate that fast radiation
chemical processes are involved in the oxygen effect.

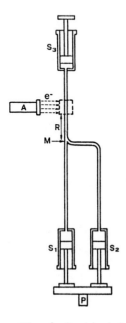

Fig. 6. Rapid mixing apparatus.

REFERENCES

1. Lilie, J., Back, G. and Hengleim, A. (1971) Ber. Bunsenges. Phys. Chem.,
    75, 458.

2. Barigelletti, F., Busi, F., Ciano, M., Concialini, V., Tubertini, O.
    and Barker, G.C., to be published.

GENERAL BIBLIOGRAPHY

M.S. Matheson and L.M. Dorfman, 1969, Pulse Radiolysis; Cambridge, Mass.:
MIT Press.

G.E. Adams, E.M. Fielden and B.D. Michael, 1975, Fast Processes in Radiation
Chemistry and Biology; Bristol: The Institute of Physics and Wiley.

P. Neta, 1976, Adv. Phys. Org. Chem. $\underline{12}$ 223-97.

J.W. Hunt, Adv. Radiat. Chem. $\underline{5}$ 185-315.

P. Wardman, Rep. Prog. Phys. $\underline{41}$ 259-302.

© 1979 Elsevier/North-Holland Biomedical Press
Radiosensitizers of Hypoxic Cells
A. Breccia, C. Rimondi and G.E. Adams eds.

MOLECULAR MECHANISM OF RADIOSENSITIZATION

R. BADIELLO and M. TAMBA

Laboratorio di Fotochimica e Radiazioni di Alta Energia (C.N.R.) - Via
Castagnoli 1, Bologna (Italy).

INTRODUCTION

The final long-term response of ionizing radiation on living systems is
the result of many processes, radiation physical, radiation chemical and
biological. The explanation of the biological effects of radiation should
start, therefore, with the initial physico-chemical changes immediately
following the absorption of energy. The study of early molecular processes
is important not only for knowledge of the mechanisms of radiobiological
damage, but also because many chemical agents, which act as modifiers of
radiation damage (i.e. radiosensitizers and radioprotectors), do so by
intervening in these initial physico-chemical reactions.

There are several ways of measuring radiation-damage, but certainly one
of the most usual can be obtained from survival curves, either of single
cells or of whole organisms.

OXYGEN AND CHEMICAL RADIOSENSITIZERS

There are many factors affecting cellular radiation sensitivity; they
derive from the intrinsic (i.e. cell cycle, metabolic state etc.) and the
environmental (i.e. oxygen content, presence of added substances etc.)
conditions of the cell. An extensive review on this subject has been
published recently[1].

Certainly the effect of oxygen in enhancing radiation damage in most
biological systems, including mammalian cells and whole organisms, has been
known for many years[2] and fundamental and clinical work on both animal and
human tumours has demonstrated the importance of anoxic regions in tumours
as a limiting factor in radiotherapy[3]. An example of the oxygen effect is
shown in fig. 1, which shows the survival curves for a radiation resistant

strain of bacteria, *E. coli B/r*. At the same dose, the surviving fraction
is considerably larger for bacteria irradiated in the absence of oxygen.
The ratio of the radiation dose given under anoxic conditions to produce
a given effect, relative to the radiation dose required to produce the same
effect under oxygenated conditions, is defined as the oxygen enhancement ratio
(OER). Relatively small concentrations of oxygen are sufficient to show the
effect both in bacterial and mammalian cells.

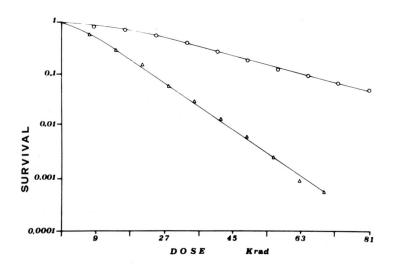

Fig. 1. Survival of E. coli B/r irradiated with X-rays in the presence of
nitrogen, O—O and of air, △—△.

Although the reactions, in which the oxygen is involved, are still far
from clear, it is well known, from experimental evidence, that they are
very fast and therefore presumably proceed on a radiation chemical, rather
than a biological level, immediately after the initial physical deposition
of energy.

It should be emphasized that the oxygen effect decreases with increasing
LET (linear energy transfer) radiation. For example charged particles, such as α
particle radiation, show a smaller oxygen effect and this physical advantage

of charged particle beams in radiotherapy of tumours containing hypoxic cells
is discussed by Professor Fowler. For high LET radiation, the primary
deposition of energy probably produces more irreversible damage which cannot
be sensitized to the same extent. This hypothesis supports the radiation-
-chemical nature of the oxygen effect and is in agreement with the mechanism of
fixation of radiation damage in a critical target of the cell.

Any chemical agent which acts similarly to oxygen on the biological
response to radiation, but is not removed by metabolism, is of potential
value in radiotherapy. This chemical approach to the problem of tumour
hypoxia seems to be, at the present, one of the more promising ones. From
a historical point of view, the first idea for improving the therapeutic
effects of tumour irradiation by means of chemical substances, was proposed in
1905 by R. Werner[4], who used a drug called enzytol, based on choline borate.
More recently, the first class of radiosensitizers studied in detail, included
compounds which bind and react with the -SH groups, since the best endogenous
and exogenous radioprotective substances contain free thiol groups. Some
positive results have been obtained with compounds affecting cellular thiol
levels, such as N-ethylmaleimide (NEM) and iodoacetic acid[5].

At the recent IAEA Panel Meeting in Vienna[6], radiosensitizers were
classified into four groups: a) hypoxic cell sensitizers, b) analogues of
DNA precursors, c) radiation-activated cytotoxic compounds, d) agents which
modify cellular regulatory processes.

Figs. 2 and 3 show the sensitizing activity on bacterial systems of agents
studied in this laboratory, including colloidal selenium[7,8] and iothalamic
acid[9,10]. In particular, Fig. 2 shows that colloidal selenium has no effect
in air but shows appreciable sensitization in the absence of oxygen. Although
colloidal selenium does not appear to have any possible practical application,
mainly because of its toxicity and instability, it exhibits a type of
radiosensitization which could contribute to an understanding of mechanisms
of anoxic sensitization. From the experimental results, it is concluded
that the sensitization is probably due to the formation, from irradiated
colloidal selenium, of short-lived species acting in processes occurring
extracellularly.

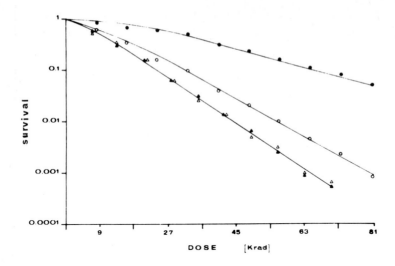

Fig. 2. Survival of E. coli B/r irradiated with X-rays in the presence of colloidal selenium; ●—● , control and O—O , colloidal selenium in nitrogen; ▲—▲, control and, △—△ , colloidal selenium in air (from R. Badiello, D. Di Maggio, M. Quintiliani and O. Sapora, Int. J. Radiat. Biol. 20, 61, 1971).

Fig. 3 shows the sensitizing effect of an iodinated contrast medium, iothalamic acid (ITA) under different experimental conditions. The sensitizing effect of ITA, as well as of other iodinated contrast media, such as diatrizoic acid (DA) and iodipamide (IP), is strong in the presence of oxygen and weak in nitrogen, as is the case with other inorganic and organic iodine--containing compounds. Short-and long-lived transient species resulting from the radiolysis of iodinated contrast media are involved in the sensitization. Even though these compounds sensitize in a way which cannot be of any interest in radiotherapy, it is important to understand their mode of action, since they could be of some potential hazard to patients referred for radiological examinations particularly at high radiation doses (i.e. in computerised tomography).

Nowadays, hypoxic cell radiosensitizers and in particular the electron-

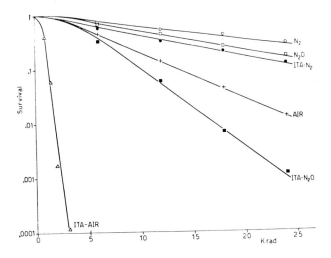

Fig. 3. Survival of E. Coli B/r irradiated with X-rays in the presence and in the absence of 10^{-2}M ioathalamic acid (ITA) in pH 5.6 buffer under different experimental conditions (from G. Simone and M. Quintiliani, Int. J. Radiat. Biol. <u>31</u>, 1, 1977).

- affinic compounds, are the most interesting ones in view of the large number of investigations carried out recently and for the promising pilot clinical studies still in progress. The Eigth Gray Conference was dedicated to"Hypoxic Cell Sensitizers in Radiobiology and Radiotherapy" as is the present Cesenatico Advanced School. The search for sensitizing, as well as for protective, compounds is no longer as haphazard as it was in the past, when biological screening was the only criterion that could be used.

It was suggested by Adams and Dewey[12] that the property of radiosensitization may be related to the electron-affinity of the sensitizer and to its conjugated structure, in which the oxidizing property is due to the stabilizing effect of electron delocalization by resonance. A number of good radiosensitizers, including dicarbonyl compounds, quinones, aromatic ketones, nitrofurans, nitroimidazoles and other miscellaneous substances were discovered, in the

main, by Adams and his Collaborators. In particular, among the few compounds
with an appreciable sensitization *in vivo* and with relatively good
pharmacological activity, the most interesting are a 5-nitroimidazole,
Metronidazole or "Flagyl" and a 2-nitroimidazole, Misonidazole. Misonidazole
is a more efficient radiosensitizer than Metronidazole. The nitro group
in position 2 of the imidazole ring interacts better with the π-electrons
of the ring than would a nitro group in position 5 and this explains the
greater electron affinity and consequently the better radiosensitization of the
2-nitroimidazole class.

MOLECULAR MECHANISMS OF RADIOSENSITIZATION

   We shall limit ourselves in discussion to some aspects of radiosensitization
at the molecular level. A possible, rough classification of sensitization
mechanisms distinguishes two principal categories of damage[13], one of radiation-
-chemical and one of biochemical nature. The former includes all fast processes
in which sensitization involves free-radicals or other short lived precursors,
while the second includes relatively slow processes between the radiosensitizers
(or its resulting radiation-induced products) and cellular components. The
biochemical processes (i.e. inhibition of cellular repair, suppression of
natural radioprotectors, change in the metabolism or in the redox state of
the cell) occur over a time scale which is much longer than that for radiation
chemical processes. Of course the distinction between the two mechanisms
is somewhat arbitrary, but the relative importance of each process can be
investigated by a comparison of the response of chemical and cellular systems
(i.e. mammalian cells). The existence of a good relationship between the
two types of response should indicate that radiation-chemical mechanisms
play a predominant role in radiosensitization. Another method for
distinguishing these different mechanisms is based on their time of action.
This can be achieved by the use of fast perturbation techniques such as
rapid mixing and pulse radiolysis. The application of basic concepts and
techniques of general radiation chemistry by Adams and his Collaborators[13]
is one of the crucial points in the study of chemical sensitizers.

Rapid mixing and pulse radiolysis are described in detail in this series
of lectures by Dr. Busi.

The rapid mixing device used in some laboratories[14-17] is designed to
mix together very rapidly, a cellular (or chemical) system with a dose
modifying agent and then to irradiate either a few milliseconds before, or
after, the mixing. In this way it has been shown that several substances,
including iodoacetamide, N-ethylmaleimide, oxygen and cysteine, modify the
radiosensitivity of bacteria even when the contact time before irradiation
is only of the order of few milliseconds thus supporting the involvement of
fast radiation chemical reactions. In particular, Adams and al.[18] showed
that radiosensitization of bacteria *Serratia marcescens* by NEM occurred very
rapidly over a time scale much shorter than that required for chemical
reaction of NEM with a sufficient amount of -SH groups to alter dramatically
cellular radiosensitivity. It was concluded that the sensitizer acts by
means of fast free radical processes.

More recently, several other sensitizers have been examined in mammalian
cells using the rapid mixing technique[17,18]. Compounds including metronidazole
and misonidazole produce significant changes in radiosensitivity after
incubation times of less than one second and this is in agreement with a
radiation-chemical mechanism.

The pulse radiolysis technique and its application in chemistry and
biology has been reviewed in many publications[19-21]. Briefly, pulse
radiolysis uses a short intense pulse of radiation to induce the initial
physical-chemical damage and fast recording techniques (i.e. absorption
kinetic spectrophotometry with oscillographic output) are used to investigate
the short-lived chemical species produced, and to follow their subsequent
reaction pathway. The most important transient species formed in water or
in aqueous solutions, are OH,H and the hydrated electron (e_{aq}^-), which are the
precursors of some of the radiation damage in biological structures.

Pulse radiolysis has been used to elucidate the molecular mechanisms of
action of many classes of radiosensitizers. Fig. 4 shows results from the
pulse radiolysis of aqueous solution of DNA containing the organic stable

82

free radical triacetoneamina-N-oxyl (TAN)[22], which is a powerful radiosensitizer.
The transient absorption of DNA radicals at about 300 nm produced by direct
attachment of OH radicals to DNA, is relatively long-lived. In the presence
of 1.5×10^{-4} M TAN, about 50% of the absorption decays rapidly over about 100
microseconds. The decay contains at least two components, a rapid one, which
decays first order with respect to TAN, and a slower one which is independent
of TAN concentration. The decay is probably due to the addition of TAN to
free radical sites produced in radiation damaged DNA.

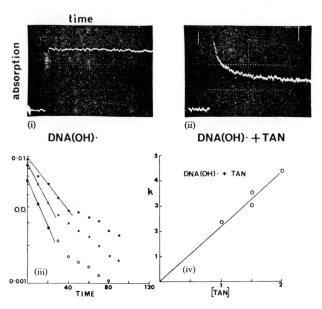

Fig. 4. Absorption decay at 310 nm after pulse radiolysis of N_2O-saturated
DNA solution (0.06 percent), (i) in the absence, (ii) in the presence of
1.4×10^{-4}M TAN. Ordinate: absorption, 1%. Abscissae: time 50 μ s per division.
Kinetic treatment of the DNA (OH) absorption decay at 310 nm, (iii)●, 10^{-4}M,
✗ 1.5×10^{-4}M; ○, 2×10^{-4}M TAN. Ordinate: optical density. Abscissa: time,
μ s. (IV) Ordinate: first order rate constant, $s^{-1} \times 10^{-4}$. Abscissa: TAN
concentration, $M \times 10^{-4}$ (from R. Willson and P.T. Emmerson, Radiation Protection
and Sensitization, H.L. Moroson and M. Quintiliani Eds., London, Taylor and
Francis Ltd (1970), p. 73).

The mechanism of action of the free radical nitroxyl compounds has been
widely investigated by Fielden and Roberts[23,24]. In particular, Nor-
-pseudopelletierine-N-oxyl (NPPN) reacts with radicals derived from thymine,

thymidylic acid and both native and denaturated DNA more rapidly than does TAN and other derivatives. This parallels its higher sensitizing efficiency.

An electron trapping model for electron-affinic sensitization was proposed by Adams[13]. The model suggests that, following direct ionization in the target molecule, thermalised electrons migrate to some electron trapping sites in the molecule. In the presence of electron-affinic compounds, electron transfer reaction from the ionized biomolecule to the radiosensitizer could occur in competition with the internal charge recombination. The final result is irreversible chemical damage to the critical molecule. This radiosensitization model has some support from studies using the pulse radiolysis technique.

Pulse radiolysis provides a method for the investigation of electron affinic properties spectrophotometrically by measuring the rate constants of electron transfer reactions from a model target free radical to potential sensitizers, or from one sensitizer to another.

For example, on irradiation of mixture of ketoderivatives (acetone, acetophenone, benzophenone, p-nitroacetophenone) Adams and co-workers[20] observed, from the sequential formation of the different transient spectra, the occurrence of a simple chain electron transfer through the four molecular structures:

$$\textit{acetone}^{-} \longrightarrow \textit{acetophenone}^{-} \longrightarrow \textit{benzophenone}^{-} \longrightarrow \textit{para-nitroacetophenone}^{-}$$

The direction of electron transfer gives the relative order of redox potentials of the compounds.

Fig. 5 shows one of the first examples of electron transfer from free radicals, derived from DNA bases, i.e. thymine, to the radiosensitizer NEM[25]. After the radiation pulse, the hydrated electrons react with thymine to produce the thymine radical, which in turn reacts with NEM by electron transfer.

Such electron transfer reactions have been shown for other electron-affinic sensitizers and in particular for the nitro-derivatives using different substrates, including purines, pyrimidines, amino acids and nucleic acids. The rate constants of these reactions are high, approaching diffusion limited

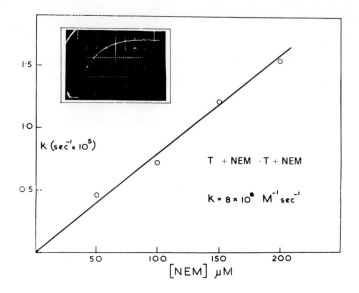

Fig. 5. The effect of NEM concentration on the rate of formation of the radical anion of NEM (NEM$^-$) by electron transfer from T$^-$. Solutions were deoxygenated and contained 5 mM thymine, 0.5 M t-butanol at pH 11.5. The rate constant for electron transfer was $8.0 \pm 0.2 \times 10^8$ M^{-1} s^{-1}. The photographic inset shows the build up of NEM$^-$ at 360 nm for a concentration of 150 μM (NEM). Each division of the abscissa represent 5 μs. (from C.L. Greenstock, G.E. Adams, R.L. Willson, Radiation Protection and Sensitization, H.L. Moroson and M. Quintiliani Eds., London, Taylor and Francis Ltd (1970), p. 65).

values[26-31], but it is difficult to relate quantitatively the values of the electron transfer rate constants with the redox potentials (or electron-affinities) of the sensitizers. An example of an electron transfer reaction will be given in the appendix.

In conclusion, the purpose of this lecture is to illustrate some significant examples of the application of radiation chemistry to chemical radiosensitization. The results demonstrate the important role played by molecular phenomena for the interpretation of mechanisms of sensitization and for the development of more active substances. Much of our information, concerning the involvement of fast processes in radiosensitization, derives from studies of simple model chemical and cellular systems carried out with fast radiation chemical

techniques. Even though the great complexity of *in vivo* systems excludes
a unique explanation of radiosensitization in molecular terms only, the
contribution of fundamental radiation chemical studies has been, and will
be, of great importance.

APPENDIX

Pulse-Radiolysis Experiment: Electron-transfer reactions between Metronidazole
("Flagyl") and nucleic acid derivatives

    The technique of pulse-radiolysis has been used to observe directly
electron-transfer reactions between nucleic acid derivatives, chosen as
model target molecules, and biological radiosensitizers in aqueous solution.

    The purpose of this laboratory experiment is to observe the electron-
-transfer processes between the electron-adducts of free DNA bases (thymine
and adenine) and the electron-affinic sensitizer metronidazole ("Flagyl"),
a 5-substituted nitroimidazole.

Metronidazole   **Thymine**   **Adenine**
   or
  "**Flagyl**"

Apparatus

    The pulse-radiolysis source is a 12 MeV Vickers Linear Accelerator[16].
Samples are irradiated in a 5 cm pathlength quartz cell with a single
electron pulse using kinetic optical absorption spectrophotometry. The dose
is monitored with the thiocyanate dosimeter. Neutral aqueous solutions
prepared with triply-distilled water are saturated with argon for about
15 min. before irradiation. Ter-butanol is used as a hydroxyl radical scavenger.

Experimental procedure

1) Measurement of the transient spectrum of the electron-adduct B^- formed
   directly by reaction of the hydrated electron during the pulse-radiolysis
   of a neutral deaerated aqueous solution containing 0.2 M t-butanol and
   1 mM base (B): thymine (Fig. 6A) or adenine (Fig. 6B).

$$e_{aq}^- + B \xrightarrow{k_1} B^-$$

$$k_1 \text{ (thymine)} = 1.7 \times 10^{10} M^{-1} s^{-1} \qquad (32)$$

$$k_1 \text{ (adenine)} = 3.0 \times 10^{10} M^{-1} s^{-1} \qquad (33)$$

2) Measurement of the transient spectrum of the electron-adduct S^- (Fig. 6A
   and 6B) formed directly by reaction of hydrated electron during the
   pulse radiolysis of a neutral deaerated aqueous solution containing 0.2
   M t-butanol and 5 μM metronidazole (S).

$$e_{aq}^- + S \xrightarrow{k_2} S^-$$

$$k_2 = 3.0 \times 10^{10} M^{-1} s^{-1} \qquad (30)$$

3) Measurement of the transient spectrum formed during the pulse-radiolysis
   of a neutral deaerated aqueous solution containing 0.2 M t-butanol,
   1 mM thymine or adenine and 5 μM metronidazole (Fig. 6A and 6B).

4) Comparison between spectra 1),2), and 3).

5) Evidence that the transient absorption bands of spectra 2) and 3) are
   similar; this means that, although almost all the hydrated electrons
   are scavenged by DNA bases, the reaction product S^- is also formed,
   showing that electron-transfer from B^- occurs:

$$B^- + S \xrightarrow{k_3} B + S^-$$

$$k_3 \text{ (thymine)} = 3.0 \times 10^9 M^{-1} s^{-1} \qquad (31)$$

$$k_3 \text{ (adenine)} = 3.3 \times 10^9 M^{-1} s^{-1}$$

6) Observation that the electron-transfer rate constants are first-order
   in metronidazole concentration and that the values are high, approaching
   diffusion-limited values.

*Figs. 2,3,4 and 5 are taken from the quoted sources with the permission of
the Publishers and of the Authors.*

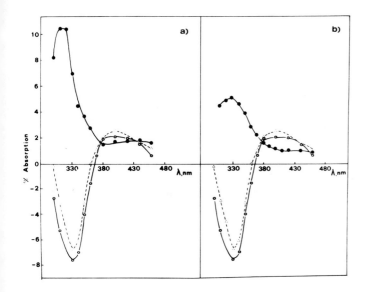

Fig. 6a. Transient absorption spectra of 1 mM adenine,●—●; 5 μm Flagyl,O—O ;
5 μM Flagyl + 1 mM adenine,△···△. Fig. 6b. Transient absorption spectra of
1 mM thymine,●—●; 5 μM Flagyl,O—O; 5 μM Flagyl + 1 mM thymine,△···△. All
spectra are recorded in deaerated aqueous solutions containing 0.2 M t-
-butanol 10 μs after the pulse. Dose ≃ 850 rad, path cell = 5 cm.

REFERENCES

1. Quintiliani, M. (1971) Ann. Ist. Super. San., 7, 647.

2. Schwarz, G. (1909) Münch. med. Wochschr, 56, 1217.

3. Van den Brenk, H.A.S. (1969) "The oxygen effect in radiation therapy",
   Current Topics in Radiation Research vol.5 North Holland Publ. Corp.
   Amsterdam, p. 197.

4. Werner, R. (1905) Münch. med. Wochschr., 52, 691.

5. Bridges, B.A. (1969) "Sensitization of organisms to radiation by sulphydryl-
   -binding agents", Adv. Radiat. Biol., vol. 3, Academic Press, New York,
   p. 123.

6. Modification of Radiosensitivity of Biological Systems, (1976) I.A.E.A.,
   Vienna.

7. Badiello,R.,Di Maggio, D., Quintiliani, M., Sapora, O. (1971) Int. J.
   Radiat. Biol. 20, 61.

8. Badiello, R., Sapora, O., Simone, G., Tamba, M. (1974) Ann. Ist. Super. Sanità, 10, 147.

9. Quintiliani, M. (1974) Advances in Chemical Radiosensitization, I.A.E.A., Vienna, International Atomic Agency, p. 87.

10. Simone, G., Quintiliani, M. (1977) Int. J. Radiat. Biol., 31, 1.

11. Br. J. Cancer, 37, Suppl. III (1978).

12. Adams, G.E., Dewey, D.L. (1963) Biochem. Biophys. Res. Comm. 12, 473.

13. Adams, G.E. (1969) "Molecular mechanisms of cellular radiosensitization and radioprotection" in Radiation Protection and Sensitization, Moroson, I.L. and Quintiliani, M. eds. (London, Taylor and Francis Ltd) p. 3.

14. Adams, G.E., Cooke, M.S., Michael, B.D. (1968) Nature, 219, 1369.

15. Brustad, T. (1968) Scand. J. Clin. Lab. Invest. Suppl. 106 (22), 31.

16. Hutton, A., Roffi, G., Martelli, A. (1974) Quad. Area Ric. Emilia-Romagna, 5, 67.

17. Whillans, D.W., Hunt, J.W. (1978) Br. J. Cancer, 37, Suppl. III, 38.

18. Adams, G.E., Michael, B.D., Asquith, I.C., Shenoy, M.A., Watts, M.E., Whillans, D.W. (1975) "Rapid mixing studies of the time scale of radiation damage in cells" in Radiation Research: Biomedical, Chemical and Physical Perspective. Nygaard, O.F., Adler, H.I., Sinclair, W.K. eds. Academic Press, New York, p. 478.

19. Matheson, M.S., Dorfman, L.M. (1969) Pulse Radiolysis, the M.I.T. Press, Cambridge, Massachusetts.

20. Adams, G.E., Baxendale, J.H., Boag, J.W., Bühler, R.E., Fielden, E.M. (1970) Pulse Radiolysis, Quad. Ric. Sci 68.

21. Badiello, R., Breccia, A. (1975) Chim. Ind., 57, 525.

22. Willson, R.L., Emmerson, P.T. (1970) "Reaction of TAN with radiation induced radicals from DNA and from deoxyribonucleotides in aqueous solution" in Radiation Protection and Sensitization, Moroson, H.L., Quintiliani, M. eds. (London, Taylor and Francis Ltd) p. 65.

23. Fielden, E.M., Roberts, P.B. (1971) Int. J. Radiat. Biol., 20, 355.

24. Roberts, P.B., Fielden, E.M. (1971) Int. J. Radiat. Biol., 20, 363.

25. Greenstock, C.L., Adams, G.E., Willson, R.L. (1970) "Electron transfer studies of nucleic acid derivatives in solutions containing radiosensitizers" in Radiation Protection and Sensitization, Moroson, H.L. and Quintiliani, M. eds. (London, Taylor and Francis Ltd) p. 65.

26. Chapman, I.D., Greenstock, C.L., Reuvers, A.P., Mc Donald, E., Dunlop, I. (1973) Radiat. Res., 53, 190.

27. Greenstock, C.L., Dunlop, I. (1973) Radiat. Res., 56, 428.

28. Greenstock, C.L., Dunlop, I. (1973) Int. J. Radiat. Biol., 23, 197.

29. Whillans, D.W., Adams, G.E. (1975) Int. J. Radiat. Biol. 28, 501.

30. Whillans, D.W., Adams, G.E., Neta, P. (1975) Radiat. Res. 62, 407.

31. Greenstock, C.L., Biaglow, I.E. Durand, R.E., Br. J. Cancer, 37 (Suppl. 3) 11.

32. Hart, E.J., Gordon, S., Thomas, J.K. (1964) J. Phys. Chem., 68, 1262.

33. Greenstock, C.L. M. Ng., J.W. Hunt, (1968) Advanc. Chem. Ser. 81, 397.

Radiosensitizers of Hypoxic Cells
A. Breccia, C. Rimondi and G.E. Adams eds.

91

THE CHEMICAL BASIS FOR THE DEVELOPMENT OF HYPOXIC CELL RADIOSENSITIZERS

PETER WARDMAN

Cancer Research Campaign Gray Laboratory, Mount Vernon Hospital, Northwood,
Middlesex HA6 2RN, England

INTRODUCTION

The clinical trials of the hypoxic cell radiosensitizers misonidazole and
metronidazole that are now under way in a number of centres are the results
of laboratory studies involving many scientists covering a period of over 20
years. These studies range from purely chemical experiments through to
measurements of radiosensitization behaviour in cultured bacterial or
mammalian cells *in vitro* and evaluation of the changes in radiation response
of tumours resulting from administering the drugs to mice prior to irradiation.

Some of the steps which have been involved in the development of radiosensitizing drugs are outlined in Figure 1. This schematic representation
is really a framework of the rationale for the development of improved hypoxic
cell radiosensitizers rather than a historical summary, since we now have the

Strategy for the development of radiosensitizers

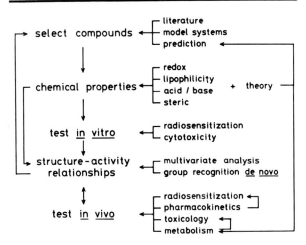

Fig. 1 - The rationale for drug development.

benefit of hindsight. Thus, whilst we now discuss the importance of differing
chemical properties in influencing radiosensitization behaviour in terms of
the Hansch equations familiar in drug design studies in medicine[1] (see
Wardman et al.[2]), it is apparent that earlier investigations which did not
involve what might be termed the Hansch vocabulary in the presentation of
data[3-6] were of great importance in the search for clinically useful
radiosensitizers.

In this paper we shall restrict ourselves to outlining some of the
chemical aspects of the rationale for drug development outlined in Figure 1.
Much of the basis for the approach is already well established in drug
research[1,7,8] and in particular the application of quantitative structure-
activity relationships (QSAR) illustrated here for radiosensitizers is that
pioneered by Hansch[1,9]. Hence this paper owes as much to medicinal chemistry
as to radiation chemistry or radiobiology. The methods and results of testing
hypoxic cell radiosensitizers both *in vitro* and *in vivo* are discussed in
detail by Dr. Stratford and Professor Fowler elsewhere in this volume. We
shall concentrate on a discussion of the chemical properties important in
radiosensitization and outline the mathematical methods used to quantify the
relative importance of different chemical properties in influencing a
biological response, whether it be sensitization behaviour or another variable
such as toxicity.

Also in this volume, Professor Adams and Dr. Dische have drawn attention
to the limitations in the concentration of radiosensitizing drug in tumours
that can be achieved after oral dosing of patients with misonidazole or
metronidazole at the highest doses tolerated. These concentrations are likely
to effect only a fraction of the maximum radiosensitizing response demonstrated
in vitro. Hence it is reasonable to search for radiosensitizers which are more
efficient than either misonidazole or metronidazole. Whether or not an
increased efficiency will always be accompanied by a parallel increase in
toxicity and hence an unchanged therapeutic ratio is the subject of much
current work, some of which is outlined in this paper.

We have presented elsewhere[2] a brief summary of the approach discussed below. Some of the more basic chemical questions have also been described in more detail previously[10].

THE SELECTION OF COMPOUNDS FOR INVESTIGATING STRUCTURE-ACTIVITY RELATIONSHIPS

Misonidazole is a 2-nitroimidazole and metronidazole a 5-nitroimidazole; both have solubilizing sidechains substituted at the nitrogen in the imidazole ring which we label as position 1 and then count other substituents clockwise round the ring (see Figure 2). Recent work at the Gray Laboratory has concentrated on evaluating many other 2-, 4- and 5-nitroimidazoles with various sidechains or substituents R^1 and R^2 which modify the chemical properties of the basic nitroimidazole structure. Earlier work (e.g. by Raleigh et al.[5] and Chapman et al.[11]) had demonstrated the efficiency of some substituted nitrobenzenes or 5-nitrofurans as radiosensitizers *in vitro* but the consequential testing *in vivo* of selected compounds from these two other classes of nitroaromatic compounds also shown in Figure 2 revealed an apparently reduced effectiveness *in vivo*[12,13]. This was probably because of metabolic inactivation and/or unfavourable pharmacokinetics in the test species[14].

More recently some other classes of nitroheteroaromatic compounds have shown activity both *in vitro* and *in vivo*, e.g. the nitropyrroles[15]. For simplicity and brevity we shall not consider these other types in the present paper. It is important to note that the essential feature of all these compounds for radiosensitization efficiency is the nitroaromatic structure.

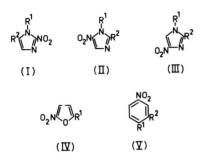

(I)   (II)   (III)

(IV)   (V)

Fig. 2 - Molecular formulae of some typical nitroaromatic radiosensitizers.

Much of what we describe here for the nitroimidazoles applies (qualitatively at least) for other series of compounds such as nitro-pyrroles, -thiazoles and -pyrazoles. These other groups of compounds could well be included in the structure-activity relationships discussed below mainly for nitroimidazoles.

QUANTITATIVE STRUCTURE-ACTIVITY RELATIONSHIPS (QSAR) IN DRUG DESIGN

One feature of the chemical structure of molecules likely to show radio-sensitizing properties is obviously, then, the nitro group substituted at a ring showing aromatic properties. (It is only obvious to us now because of the great deal of work which led to the identification[16,17] of 4-nitroaceto-phenone as an efficient sensitizer and many investigations since; our purpose here is to outline the basis for future work and not present a historical review).

Earlier classes of compounds which were identified as radiosensitizers included, e.g. conjugated ketones[4] and quinones[18,4]. However, the more powerful oxidizing agents such as the nitro compounds seem much more efficient and clearly warrant the detailed examination of QSAR now in progress. Within the general class of nitro compounds, we have to identify other chemical features of the molecules which may influence their biological behaviour. We could attempt to do this by trying to recognize the particular fragments or groups in molecules, the inclusion of which seem to have a connection with activity. This 'group recognition' approach is illustrated by the 'Free-Wilson' model[19]. In the present work a simpler and more successful approach is to identify and quantify those physico-chemical properties of the molecule as a whole which can be correlated with biological activity: the Hansch approach[1,9].

Nitro compounds are well-known for their ease of chemical reduction and hence the redox properties of the molecule would be one suitable area to investigate. The distribution and rate of passage of a molecule across any biological phase boundary, e.g. in aqueous phases separated by a lipoidal membrane will be influenced by equilibrium partition properties which vary according to the lipophilicity of the molecule as a whole. Further, charged compounds generally cross biological membranes much less efficiently than uncharged molecules and the presence of ionizable groups or proton acceptor sites in the molecule may have important consequences, especially in the pharmacokinetics of drug absorption and elimination *in vivo*[20].

To attempt to derive successful QSAR's using the Hansch approach and illustrated below using a mathematical model, we have, then, to identify and quantify (i) the appropriate biological responses such as radiosensitization efficiency, cytotoxicity, etc. and (ii) appropriate chemical properties such as electronic or redox properties (electron affinity), lipophilicity and the pK_a's of acid-base equilibria. We might note that, whilst if we were to begin to design a radiosensitizing molecule'from scratch' today, we would naturally investigate the importance of redox properties, historically the importance of electron affinity in radiosensitization was identified[3] before the Hansch approach became well-known[21].

REDUCTION POTENTIALS AS A GUIDE TO ELECTRON AFFINITY

Adams and Dewey noted 15 years ago[3] that some compounds S which radio-sensitize hypoxic cells react rapidly with hydrated electrons (e_{aq}^-, very reactive species produced when aqueous solutions are irradiated):

$$S + e_{aq}^- \rightleftharpoons S^- \tag{1}$$

The *rates* at which e_{aq}^- react with nitroaromatic radiosensitizers are in fact all very similar (e.g. Whillians et al.[22]). However, we can express the affinity of S for e_{aq}^- or define the stability of S^- in terms of the energy liberated when e_{aq}^- and S react together. This can be expressed in volts to establish a quantitative scale related to electron affinity.

Reaction (1) does not only occur when water is irradiated: electron-attachment to S (reduction of S) can be achieved at the surface of an electrode in solution if a suitable potential is applied. Thus electro-chemical methods are frequently used to measure reduction potentials[23]. These include polarography and cyclic voltametry, methods described elsewhere in these proceedings by Dr. Roffia. Some reduction potentials for quinones and other non-nitro compounds have been discussed elsewhere[10], where we differentiate between one-electron reduction and overall reduction, e.g.

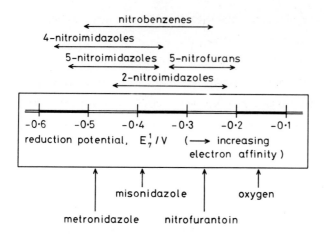

Fig. 3 - One-electron reduction potentials (E_7^1) of radiosensitizers at pH 7 in water at $\sim$ 298 K.

4-electron reduction of a nitro compound to give a hydroxylamine. The one-electron potential, E is related to polarographic half-wave potentials obtained both in water (see Wardman[10]) and an aprotic solvent[24].

Figure 3 summarises the most important results we have obtained using the pulse radiolysis method to measure the values of E of nitro radio-sensitizers.[25,26] The general method and applications of pulse radiolysis have been reviewed recently.[27,28] More electron-affinic compounds have more positive reduction potentials, i.e. are towards the right of the Figure. The reference or 'zero' on the scale is the potential for the reduction of H^+ at pH 0. The range of potentials for a given class of compounds (e.g. for 2-nitroimidazoles from ca. -240 to -450 mV) reflects the influence of groups in addition to NO_2 substituted in the imidazole ring (see below).

From Figure 3 we conclude: (i) oxygen is more electron-affinic than all the nitro compounds shown; (ii) the relative order of decreasing electron-affinity is, in general: 5-nitrofurans; 2-nitroimidazoles; 5-nitroimidazoles; 4-nitroimidazoles; (iii) there is some overlap between classes so we can obtain 2-nitroimidazoles as electron-affinic as nitrofurans.

We have demonstrated elsewhere[10,26,29] the effects of substitution of electron-withdrawing or -donating groups into the imidazole ring. Some

examples are illustrated below. To illustrate the magnitude of the effects
of such substitution we can compare the difference in E between misonidazole
and metronidazole (ca. 100 mV) with the increase in potential of ca. 150 mV
resulting from substitution of the CHO group in *either* the 5-position in a
2-nitroimidazole[26] *or* the 2 position of a 5-nitroimidazole (Clarke and
Wardman, unpublished).

ALTERATION OF THE LIPOPHILICITY OF NITROIMIDAZOLES

     As a quantitative guide to the lipophilicity of a molecule we define a
partition coefficient P, which is the ratio of the equilibrium concentrations
of a compound in the lipid phase (e.g. octanol) and aqueous phase (e.g. pH
7.4 buffer) when distributed in such a biphasic system. The higher the value
of P, the more lipophilic the compound. Often, values of *log* P are tabulated[30],
for reasons which will become apparent.

     The magnitude of P in, e.g. substituted nitroimidazoles will be influenced
by (i) the position of the NO_2 group in the ring and (ii) other substituents.
For nitroimidazoles with identical sidechains, R^1 at N-1 ($R^1 \neq H$) the
lipophilicities P for 2-, 4- and 5-nitrosubstitution are in the approximate
ratio: 1:0.5:1.8 respectively. For a series of 1-methyl-2-nitroimidazoles
substituted at C-5 the lipophilicities vary as illustrated in Figure 4.

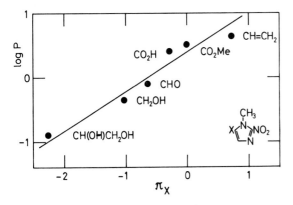

Fig. 4 - Correlation of measured values of the octanol: water partition
         coefficient P with the Hansch π_X substituent constant.

Here measured values of log P are plotted against a substituent parameter π_X, defined by Fujita et al.[31] as the difference between log P for, e.g. a substituted benzene and log P for benzene itself (X = H). We see that groups with fairly similar effects on lipophilicity may have markedly different effects on redox properties (e.g. CHO, CH_2OH). A similar relationship between log P and π_X was found for analogues of misonidazole[2]. Thus if we measure P for 2 or 3 derivatives in a series we may be able to predict the lipophilicities of other derivatives by use of tables[32] of the lipophilicity function π_X.

DEPENDENCE OF RADIOSENSITIZATION EFFICIENCY UPON REDUCTION POTENTIAL

Dr. Stratford discusses elsewhere in these Proceedings the methods used to measure radiosensitization efficiency and cytotoxicity *in vitro*. It is convenient to compare the sensitizing efficiencies of different compounds in terms of the concentrations required to achieve a particular sensitizer enhancement ratio (SER). The concentration range over which measurements may be made *in vitro* will be determined either by the solubility limit in aqueous medium or interference from the cytotoxic action of the compounds during the minimum time required for carrying out the sensitization experiment. An illustration of the type of data[33] obtained is shown in the curves of SER vs. concentration for the 3 compounds in Figure 5. It is convenient[33] to read off the concentrations required to reach an SER of 1.6, $C_{1.6}$ as an arbitrary though useful definition of sensitization efficiency. For the compounds illustrated in Figure 5, we note that this concentration range covers a factor of about 500. Also, the curves are rather shallow - we may need around 2-3 times as much compound to increase the SER from e.g. 1.4 to 1.6, especially for the less efficient sensitizers[29].

In Figure 6 we have plotted data[29] for the radiosensitization efficiency of many nitro compounds vs. the reduction potential E. The use of the logarithm of the reciprocal concentration (-log C = log 1/C) can be justified from descriptions of other model systems[21]. Figure 6 shows data for 4 different classes of nitroheterocyclic compound. We have demonstrated elsewhere[29] that both oxygen and a quinone have radiosensitization efficiencies

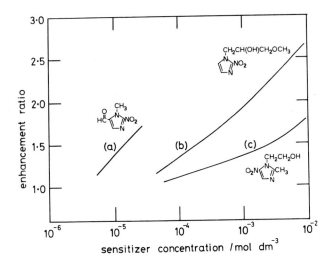

Fig. 5 - Sensitizer enhancement ratios (SER) obtained for 3 nitroimidazoles using the Chinese Hamster cell line V79-379A *in vitro*.

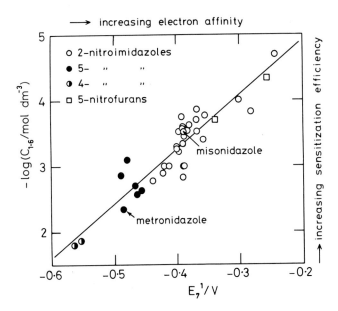

Fig. 6 - Correlation of the radiosensitization efficiency (concentration required for SER = 1.6 *in vitro*) with the reduction potential E.

similar to what we would predict for a nitroaromatic compound of the same one-electron reduction potential, illustrating that although the nitro group is one way to achieve efficient sensitization, it is not an essential property of a hypoxic cell radiosensitizer.

REDOX DEPENDENCE OF CYTOTOXICITY IN VITRO

From Figure 6 one might conclude that it would be a simple matter to develop compounds more *efficient* than misonidazole or metronidazole. Indeed it is: one simply looks for molecules with higher reduction potentials. Unfortunately, the search for compounds of a higher *therapeutic ratio* is less straightforward. We have already published[34] a graph rather similar to Figure 6 except for the replacement of radiosensitization efficiency as the biological response by a measure (in concentration terms) of the toxicity of the nitro compounds towards oxic cells *in vitro*. The slope of these two graphs are similar, i.e. the dependence upon reduction potential of both radiosensitization efficiency and cytotoxicity towards normal (oxic) cells is similar. Hence (as a broad generalization) more efficient sensitizers are likely to be more toxic. We do not know whether cytotoxicity *in vitro* closely parallels the observed dose-limiting physiological response *in vivo*.

INFLUENCE OF NON-REDOX PROPERTIES ON RADIOSENSITIZATION *IN VITRO*

The straight-line relationship in Figure 6 can be represented by the equation:

$$- \log C = 6.54 + 8.21 \ (E/V) \tag{2}$$

and regression analysis (least-squares fit) of the data[29] yields the statistical parameters: n = 38, r = 0.923 and ev = 0.847. (Here n is the number of data sets, r the correlation coefficient and ev the explained variance). The value ev = 0.847 indicates that $\sim$ 85 percent of the behaviour of the dependent variable -log C can be explained by the variation in the independent variable E. The scatter in Figure 6 arises from two sources: (i) random error in measurement of SER as a function of concentration, which may be appreciable because of the relatively 'flat' response of increasing

SER with concentration, especially at low SER, and (ii) properties which influence -log C. The latter may include additional independent variables (chemical properties) and unknown systematic errors in measurement such as those which might arise if the cell growth medium is changed over a long period of investigation.

We know[29] that the measured lipophilicities (P) of the molecules whose behaviour is described by Figure 6 range from 0.05 to > 100. To test whether part of the unexplained variance in -log C arises from the additional variable P (as log P)[1] we repeat the least-squares analysis with the two independent variables E and log P. The technique of multiple linear regression[35] is used to fit the data, resulting in the equation:

$$- \log C = 6.52 + 8.16 \ (E/V) + 0.04 \ \log P \qquad (3)$$

with n = 38, r = 0.924 and ev = 0.845. Note the slight *decrease* in explained variance, i.e. inclusion of log P in the equation has not helped in fitting the data. Indeed, the standard error of the coefficient for log P (0.06) is greater than the coefficient itself (0.04). This means that our data has not demonstrated *any* influence of partition properties upon sensitizing efficiency[29].

A similar analysis[34] in which aerobic cytotoxicity was used as the biological response led to a similar failure to demonstrate any influence of P on cytotoxicity *in vitro*. Further expansion of equation (3) to allow for the possibility that any influence of P was quadratic (curved or passing through a maximum) was not helpful[29,34].

POSSIBLE IMPORTANCE OF PARTITION PROPERTIES *IN VIVO*

The apparent lack of importance of partition properties *in vitro* may not be a reliable guide to the behaviour *in vivo* of nitroimidazoles differing in their lipophilicities. One example in the literature[36] to which we recently drew attention[2] is the use of substituted 5-nitroimidazoles as antitrichomonal agents *in vivo*. Butler et al.[36] measured the oral dose required to cure 50 percent of mice infected with *Trichomonas foetus*, using a series of 5-nitroimidazoles rather similar to metronidazole except that the OH group in the latter was replaced by a CN group (see Figure 7). The CH$_3$ group which is substituted in the 2-position in metronidazole was changed to H, CH$_3$, C$_2$H$_5$, C$_3$H$_7$ etc., so that as the size of the 2-alkyl substituent increased, the lipophilicity P increased in a regular manner. Such changes would have little effect on E, which may be assumed constant and equation (3) modified to exclude E, but expanded to a quadratic, i.e. the equation of a parabola:

$$- \log C = -1.05 + 0.94 \log P - 2.92 (\log P)^2 \qquad (4)$$

In this example the variance in log P explained $\sim$ 74 percent of the variance of -log C, and differentiation of equation (4) gives the value P = 1.5 for optimum activity in this system.

This dependence on P of a biological response *in vivo* may include contributions from at least two factors: (i) a dependence upon P of the activity towards the trichomonad which may occur at the cellular level and

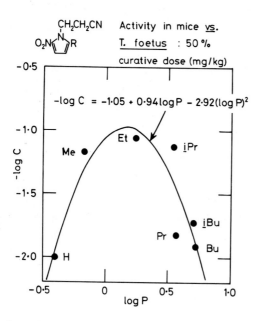

Fig. 7 - Effect of lipophilicity of some 5-nitroimidazoles on curative dose *p.o.* in mice, *vs. Trichomonas foetus*. Data from Butler et al. (1967)

is seen even *in vitro*[37], and (ii) an effect of variations in P in influencing the concentration of the compound at the active site by pharmacological responses such as the absorption, distribution and elimination of the compound. Further work is needed to see whether we have a qualitatively similar, although probably less marked influence of P upon radiosensitization *in vivo*.

THE HAMMETT SIGMA CONSTANT AS AN ALTERNATIVE TO REDUCTION POTENTIAL FOR STRUCTURE-ACTIVITY RELATIONSHIPS

Other measures of redox or electron-accepting properties may be valuable in QSAR. The Hammett σ (sigma) constant is, in fact, used more frequently than E in Hansch correlations[1]. Hammett[38] defined a substituent constant σ_X as the difference in pK_a between benzoic acid and benzoic acid substituted with the group X. The more electron-affinic the group X, the higher the value of σ_X.

Clarke and Wardman (unpublished) showed that the change in E in 1-methyl 2-nitroimidazoles substituted with the group X in the 5 position could be related to the Hammett σ value of the substituent. Some of the data is illustrated in Figure 8. The more electron-withdrawing the substituent X, the higher the value of its Hammett σ and the greater the increase in E resulting from substitution.

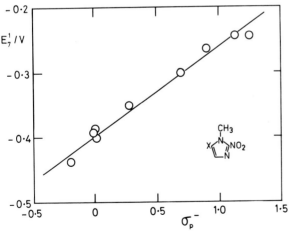

Fig. 8 - Correlation of one-electron reduction potential, E with Hammett σ constant for some 1-methyl-2-nitroimidazoles.

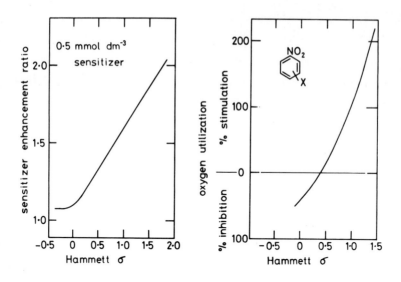

Fig. 9 - Structure-activity relationships for substitued nitrobenzenes. (a) Radiosensitization; (b) Effect on respiration *in vitro*.

Within a given series of compounds, it is not surprising therefore that the Hammett σ constant can be interchanged with E in structure-activity relationships. Two examples of this use of σ have been reported for different aspects of the use of radiosensitizers, and are illustrated in Figure 9. The left-hand plot relates the SER (for radiosensitization *in vitro*) using a fixed concentration of nitrobenzenes substituted with the group X to the Hammett σ value of the substituent[5]. The right-hand graph relates   to the effect of similar compounds on cell respiration *in vitro*[39].

Thus substituted nitrobenzenes which are more electron-affinic: (i) give higher values of SER and (ii) increase the respiration rate of Chinese Hamster cells *in vitro*. Higly electron-affinic compounds could conceivably help to create hypoxic areas *in vivo*. However, we know for example that the electron-affinity of nitrobenzene itself (σ_X = 0) is similar to that of metronidazole[25,26] and it seems likely that metronidazole and misonidazole have a relatively small influence on respiration.

OTHER CHEMICAL PROPERTIES WHICH MAY BE IMPORTANT IN INFLUENCING
RADIOSENSITIZATION OF TOXICITY

Lipid-rich or other biological membranes generally allow only uncharged molecules to pass with ease, so that ionization behaviour will be important in influencing, for example, the pharmacokinetic properties of drugs[20] in addition to influencing molecular interactions such as a drug-protein binding. A simple illustration of the consequences of acid-base behaviour is shown in Figure 10, which is modified from a standard text[20]. We consider the ionization of e.g. a nitroimidazole with a side chain at N-1 terminating in a base, so that the pK_a of the conjugate acid is 8.4:

$$O_2N-\emptyset-(CH_2)_n \; NR^1R^2H^+ \rightleftharpoons O_2N-\emptyset-(CH_2)_n \; NR^1R^2 + H^+$$

where $\emptyset$ represents the imidazole nucleus. For convenience we can simplify this equation to:

$$BH^+ \rightleftharpoons B + H^+$$

In a biologica- fluid such as plasma with pH = 7.4, the ratio of $[B]$ to $[BH^+]$ will be given by the Henderson-Hasselbach equation:

$$[B]/[BH^+] = 10^{(pH-pK_a)}$$

i.e. will be [B] : $[BH^+]$ = 1:10 if pK_a = 8.4 and pH = 7.4 (where square brackets denote concentration). However, in urine with pH = 5.4, for example,

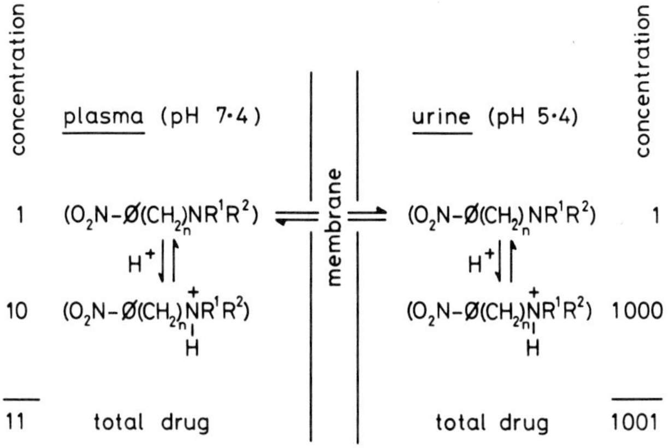

Fig. 10 - Distribution of a weak base with pK_a = 8.4 between plasma and urine.

106

$[B]:[BH^+]$ will be 1 : 1000. If the membrane is permeable only to B and not to BH^+, then the ratio of total drug concentration ($[B] + [BH^+]$) across the membrane at equilibrium will be of the order plasma: urine $\simeq$ 1:100. We can see that ionization equilibria can greatly influence the concentration gradients important in drug excretion. This example is a hypothetical illustration as we have extensive information only *in vitro* concerning the use of nitroimidazoles with ionizable groups in the sidechain. However, it illustrates the rationale behind current work.

CONCLUSIONS

We have had some success in applying the concepts of QSAR to radio-sensitization by nitro compounds and have an extensive experience of the redox chemistry and physicochemical properties of the compounds. The framework for the expansion of effort in this area, which seems justified from the encouraging clinical work discussed by Dr. Dische and Professor Rimondi at this Conference, is therefore clear. We are hopeful that increased national and international collaboration will identify compounds with an improvement in therapeutic ratio over misonidazole and metronidazole.

ACKNOWLEDGEMENTS

This work is supported by the Cancer Research Campaign. The author is indebted to Professors A. Breccia and C. Rimondi for their invitation to participate in this Conference. The Gray Laboratory work summarised in this paper is the result of a team effort spread over a number of years also involving collaboration with colleagues in the pharmaceutical industry: the author is privileged to be their spokesman on this occasion.

REFERENCES

1. Hansch, C. (1971) in Drug Design, Ariëns, E.J. ed., Academic Press, New York, pp. 271-342.

2. Wardman, P., Clarke, E.D., Flockhart, I.R. and Wallace, R.G. (1978) Br. J. Cancer, 37, Suppl. III, 1-5.

3. Adams, G.E. and Dewey, D.L. (1963) Biochem. Biophys. Res. Commun., 12, 473-477.

4. Adams, G.E. and Cooke, M.S. (1969) Int. J. Radiat. Biol., 15, 457-471.

5. Raleigh, J.A., Chapman, J.D., Borsa, J., Kremers, W. and Reuvers, A.P. (1973) Int. J. Radiat. Biol., 23, 377-387.

6. Simic, M. and Powers, E.L. (1974) Int. J. Radiat. Biol., 26, 87-90.

7. Purcell, W.R., Bass, G.E. and Clayton, J.M. (1973) Strategy of Drug Design: A Guide to Biological Activity, Wiley, New York.

8. Keverling Buisman, J.A., ed. (1977) Biological Activity and Chemical Structure, Elsevier, Amsterdam.

9. Gould, R.F., ed., (1972) Biological Correlations - The Hansch Approach, Adv. Chem. Ser. 114, American Chemical Society, Washington, D.C.

10. Wardman, P. (1977) Curr. Top. Radiat. Res. Q., 11, 347-398.

11. Chapman, J.D., Reuvers, A.P. and Borsa, J. (1973) Brit. J. Radiol., 46, 623-630.

12. Denekamp, J. and Michael, B.D. (1972) Nature New Biol., 239, 21-24.

13. Rauth, A.M. and Kaufman, K. (1975) Brit. J. Radiol., 48, 209-220.

14. Paul, H.E.and Paul, M.F. (1964) In Experimental Chemotherapy, Vol. 2, part 1, Schnitzer, R.J. and Hawking, F., eds., Academic Press, New York, pp. 307-370.

15. Raleigh, J.A., Chapman, J.D., Reuvers, A.P., Biaglow, J.E., Durand, R.E. and Rauth, A.M. (1978) Brit. J. Cancer, 37, Suppl. III, 6-10.

16. Adams, G.E., Asquith, J.C., Dewey, D.L., Foster, J.L., Michael, B.D. and Willson, R.L. (1971) Int. J. Radiat. Biol., 19, 575-585.

17. Chapman, J.D., Webb, R.G. and Borsa, J. (1971) Int. J. Radiat. Biol., 19, 561-574.

18. Mitchell, J.S. and Marrian, D.H. (1965) In Biochemistry of Quinones, Morton, R.A., ed., Academic Press, London, pp. 503-541.

19. Free, S.M., Jr., and Wilson, J.W. (1964) J. Med. Chem., 7, 395.

20. La Du, B.N., Mandel, H.G. and Way, E.L., eds. (1971) Fundamentals of Drug Metabolism and Drug Disposition, Williams & Wilkins, Baltimore, pp. 3-62.

21. Hansch, C. and Fujita, T. (1964) J. Amer. Chem. Soc., 86, 1616-1626.

22. Whillians, D.W., Adams, G.E. and Neta, P. (1975) Radiat. Res., 62, 407-421.

23. Clark, W.M. (1960) Oxidation-Reduction Potentials of Organic Systems, Williams and Wilkins, Baltimore.

24. Breccia, A., Roffia, S. and Berrilli, G. (1978) Int. J. Radiat. Biol., in the press.

25. Meisel, D. and Neta, P. (1975) J. Amer. Chem. Soc., 97, 5198-5203.

26. Wardman, P. and Clarke, E.D. (1976) J. Chem. Soc. Faraday Trans. I, 72, 1377-1390.

27. Baxendale, J.H. and Rodgers, M.A.J. (1978) Chem. Soc. Revs., 7, 235-263.

28. Wardman, P. (1978) Rep. Prog. Phys., 41, 259-302.

29. Adams, G.E., Clarke, E.D., Flockhart, I.R., Jacobs, R.S., Sehmi, D.S., Stratford, I.J., Wardman, P., Watts, M.E., Parrick, J., Wallace, R.G. and Smithen, C.E. (1978) Int. J. Radiat. Biol., in the press.

30. Leo, A., Hansch, C. and Elkins, D. (1971) Chem. Rev., 71, 525-616.

31. Fujita, T., Iwasa, J. and Hansch, C. (1964) J. Amer. Chem. Soc., 86, 5175-5180.

32. Hansch, C., Leo, A., Unger, S.H., Kim, H.K., Nikaitani, D. and Lien, E.J. (1973) J. Med. Chem., 16, 1207-16.

33. Adams, G.E., Flockhart, I.R., Smithen, C.E., Stratford, I.J., Wardman, P. and Watts, M.E. (1976) Radiat. Res., 67, 9-20.

34. Adams, G.E., Clarke, E.D., Gray, P., Jacobs, R.S., Stratford, I.J., Wardman, P., Watts, M.E., Parrick, J., Wallace, R.G. and Smithen, C.E. (L978) Int. J. Radiat. Biol., in the press.

35. Draper N.R. and Smith, H. (1966) Applied Regression Analysis, Wiley, New York.

36. Butler, K., Howes, H.L., Lynch, J.E. and Pirie, D.K. (1967) J. Med. Chem. 10, 891-897.

37. Chien, Y.W. and Mizuba, S.S. (1978) J. Med. Chem. 21, 374-380.

38. Hammett, L.P. (1970) Physical Organic Chemistry, 2nd edition, McGraw-Hill, New York, pp. 347-390.

39. Biaglow, J.E. and Durand, R.E. (1976) Radiat. Res. 65, 529-539.

© 1979 Elsevier/North-Holland Biomedical Press
Radiosensitizers of Hypoxic Cells
A. Breccia, C. Rimondi and G.E. Adams eds.

CELLULAR RADIOSENSITIZATION: PRINCIPLES AND METHODS OF STUDY

IAN J. STRATFORD

Physics Division, Institute of Cancer Research, Sutton, Surrey, U.K.

1. INTRODUCTION

The development and use of oxygen mimetic radiosensitizing drugs is arguably one of the major contributions of radiobiology and radiation chemistry to the treatment of the cancer patient by radiotherapy. This progress is based on fundamental physical chemical and radiation chemical observations, which allowed the testing of hypoxic cell radiosensitizing drugs in spores and vegetative bacteria and finally *in vitro* mammalian cell systems. The demonstration of radiosensitization of hypoxic mammalian cells *in vitro* promptly stimulated the *in vivo* testing of suitable compounds which has resulted in the clinical evaluation of the best compounds developed to date vis. misonidazole and metronidazole.

This chapter takes a cursory look at the *in vitro* mammalian cell methods used to evaluate the potential of any particular compound for use as a radiosensitizer. This includes an examination of the radiosensitizing effect on various *in vitro* cell systems together with the effects of different qualities of radiation. The methods used to equate the sensitizing efficiency of any compounds with the physical chemical properties of that compound (i.e., the formulation of structure activity relationships) are discussed. Finally the toxicity of potential radiosensitizers is reviewed, and this includes the discussion of the differential hypoxic cell toxicity seen with the nitro aromatic radiosensitizers and speculation as to the possible role of nitroaromatic compounds in combination chemoterapy.

2. TECHNIQUES

In vitro mammalian cell work can be carried out with any of a wide variety of established cell lines of rodent or human origin. Alternatively, a primary cell line might be used, this is one obtained by explanation and which is only able to undergo a certain number of passages *in vitro*. Radiobiological techniques are available to study the effects of radiosensitizing drugs on ascynchronous populations of exponentially growing or plateau phase cells. Alternatively, the development of the *in vitro* spheroid system, which is a multicellular aggregate, provides a tumour model of undoubted

110

value. Other *in vitro* techniques available generally are used in concert
with *in vivo* methods and these include, for example, treatment *in vivo*
and assay *in vitro* or alternatively, treatment *in vitro* and assay *in vivo*[1,2].
For all these techniques the *in vitro* end-point is cell survival and this
is defined as the ability of a single cell to form a colony (or undergo
a certain number of divisions) within a given time after treatment.

2.1. Single cell populations

With the established cell lines now available it is possible to treat
cells while they are attached to a support, or when the cells are in
suspension. In order to investigate the effects of O_2 and hypoxic cell
sensitizing drugs on the radiation sensitivity of cells, systems have been
devised to rigorously control the O_2 status of the cells being irradiated.
For cells attached, or in mono-layer, the support is generally glass
(petri-dish or cover slip); plastic is not suitable for irradiations under
hypoxic conditions[3]. A vessel for irradiating cells in mono-layer under
controlled gas conditions is shown in Fig. 1a and 1b[4]. The vessel, constructed

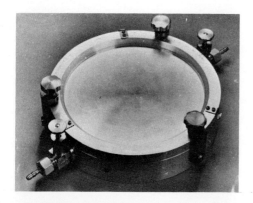

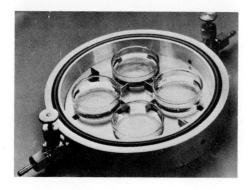

Fig. 1a and b: Aluminium-steel
vessels for irradiating mammalian
cells attached to glass.

of an aluminium/steel alloy, has positions for four petri dishes containing
known numbers of cells. The lid has a central area 4mm thick through which
the radiation beam enters and the lid is tightly clamped onto an O-ring
seal by means of three thumb screws. Two needle valves connected to the
body of the vessel enable cultures to be purged with gas (for cells covered
by 2ml of medium in a 5cm petri dish 1 hour is sufficient for equilibration
with the flushing gas). The inlet and outlet ports are then sealed and
the samples are then ready for irradiation. Immediately after irradiation
the petri dishes are removed from the apparatus and the medium removed and
replaced with fresh medium. The cells are then incubated for a sufficient
time to allow colony formation and the number of cells surviving a given
radiation treatment can be determined from the ratio of the number of colonies
counted after incubation to the number of cells originally plated.

Cells in suspension can be irradiated in a vessel similar to that illustrated
in Fig. 2[5]. This is a borosilicate glass or pyrex vessel fitted with a

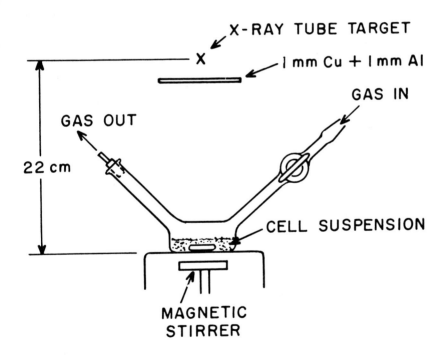

Fig. 2. Borosilicate glass vessel for irradiating cells in suspension.

gas inlet/outlet system. Positioned ready for irradiation, the stirred suspension of cells can be deaerated by flowing N_2 over the surface of the suspension (a 20ml suspension stirred at 200 rpm in a 5cm diameter vessel gassed with N_2 at a rate of 500ml/min should be rendered radiobiologically hypoxic within 30 minutes). N_2 flow and stirring should be continued throughout the irradiation. After exposure to desired radiation doses, aliquots can be withdrawn via the gas exit port for the determination of the number of surviving cells.

An alternative method for treating cells in suspension has been described by Hall and his co-workers[6]. Briefly, this involves placing an aliquot of cells a long-necked glass ampule, which can be sealed and irradiated. For hypoxic experiments N_2 is passed into the ampule via a long cannula to displace the air above the cell suspension, then with the N_2 still flowing the cannula was partially withdrawn and the ampule heat sealed. After sealing the ampulse were agitated at 27°C to allow the cells to remove any remaining O_2 by respiration. After treatment the ampule may be broken and the number of surviving cells determined.

Typical of the data generated by any of these techniques is that shown in Fig. 3, results are shown for irradiation in oxygen, nitrogen and in various concentrations of the hypoxic cell sensitizer TAN (Triacetoneamine N-oxyl)[5]. Cell survival is plotted as a function of radiation dose and it can be seen that O_2 increases the radiation sensitivity of these cells, and the oxygen enhancement ratio, defined as the ratio of the slopes of the exponential portions of the survival curves in N_2 and O_2 is 2.8. The enhancement of radiation response by the presence of TAN under hypoxic conditions is 1.33 and 1.54 for 1mM + 10mM TAN respectively. These enhancements are determined by comparing the slope of the survival curve obtained in the presence of sensitizer with that seen in hypoxia alone. For TAN and all the sensitizers discussed in this chapter sensitization only occurs under hypoxic conditions, there is no sensitization in air.

The tecniques described above have been used to determine the ability of many compounds to sensitize hypoxic cells to the lethal effects of ionizing radiation. The amount of sensitization is independent of the techniques used, appears to be independent of whether the cell is in exponential or stationary phase and also is independent of the cell line used (for further discussion see section 4/1 and Fig. 8).

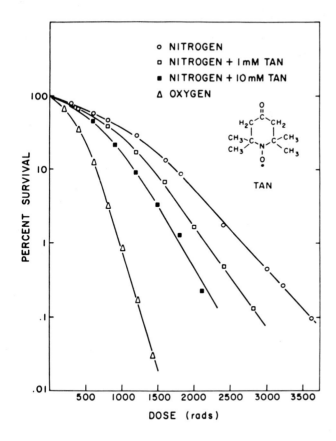

Fig. 3. Survival curves for Chinese hamster CH_2B_2 cells irradiated in air, nitrogen and in the presence of various concentrations of the sensitizer TAN under hypoxic conditions.

2.2. Spheroids[7]

These are multicellular aggregates. Some cell lines maintained in suspension culture in a well defined growth medium will aggregate into small clumps of cells then grow by cell division to multicellular structures or spheroids as large as 10^6 cells. As the spheroid enlarges the internal cells become depleted in nutrients and oxygen, which leads to the development of non-cycling and hypoxic populations.

Autoradiographs of cross-sections of spheroids labelled with H^3 thymidine have shown that these non-cycling populations begin to develop in spheroids > 250 µm diameter. With larger spheroids a distinct central necrotic area

114

is apparent, so that the *in vitro* spheroid can provide a convenient model of many solid tumours for radiation and/or drug studies.

After treatment with drugs, radiation or any other modality the spheroid is reduced to a single cell suspension using trypsin and mechanical agitation. The viability of these cells can then be estimated by using conventional colony-forming criteria.

Irradiation of the *in vitro* spheroid is essentially an irradiation of a mixed population of hypoxic and aerobic cells. This is illustrated in Fig. 4, where the open circles represent the radiation response of mono-layer cells in air and the crosses the radiation response of the intact spheroid.

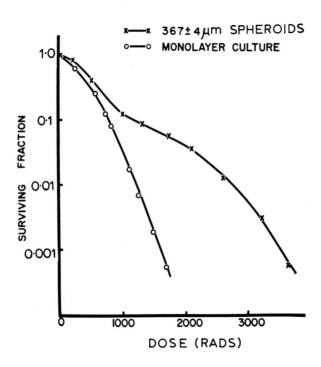

Fig. 4. Survival curves for V79-171B cells irradiated in air as monolayer cultures or as spheroids.

Clearly, the survival curve for the spheroid is biphasic. The initial portion of the curve corresponds well with the aerobic mono-layer survival curve and is taken to show the decrease in survival of the aerobic cells in the spheroid. The second phase of the survival curve represents the response of the more radiation resistant hypoxic cells, which dominate the response after the major proportion of the aerobic cells are killed.

The radiation response of intact spheroids in the presence of an electron-affinic sensitizer is shown in Fig. 5. The sensitizer used was nifuroxime,

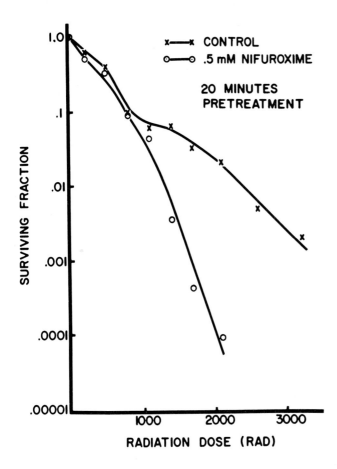

Fig. 5. Survival curves for spheroids irradiated in the presence and absence of the hypoxic cell radiosensitizer nifuroxime.

one of a series of nitrofurans shown to be very efficient radiosensitizers of cells in mono-layer[8]. The survival curve obtained for spheroids irradiated in the absence of drug is indicated by the crosses in the Figure i.e., the biphasic curve, as described above. However, in the presence of nifuroxime the hypoxic portion of the spheroid response curve is removed, yielding data (the open circles) closely resembling that seen for all the cells being fully oxygenated.

This work was thought to be an indication that an electron-affinic sensitizer could penetrate a dense cell mass to the regions in an *in vitro* tumour model where hypoxic cells were located and, once there, sensitize these cells to the lethal effects of radiation.

3. ROUTINE STUDIES ON POTENTIAL HYPOXIC CELL RADIOSENSITIZERS

In the preceding section some of the *in vitro* cell survival techniques used for determining the effects of sensitizers on the hypoxic cell radiation response were described. In this way compounds representative of many different classes have been evaluated and the nitroimidazoles, misonidazole and metronidazole have subsequently proceeded to *in vivo* testing and clinical trials.

The rationale behind the search for more efficient radiosensitizers than misonidazole and metronidazole is described by Wardman in this volume and in reference 9. At this time, synthesis and development of new compounds is underway in many centres throughout the world and generally, *in vitro* testing is the first step in the evaluation of a compound as a radiosensitizer. This testing is carried out firstly by determining the toxicity of the compound. This is done by exposing cells to the compound for a time sufficient to carry out a subsequent radiation experiment, usually about 2 hours. When this "experimental toxicity" is known radiation survival curves for cells in the presence of various non-toxic concentrations of drug under hypoxic conditions can be obtained. Typical data is shown in figure 6 for two newly synthesized compounds (see ref 10 for details), clearly at the concentrations used, RGW 609 (open squares) is a better sensitizer than RGW 611 (closed squares). From these survival curves enhancement ratios can be determined and the values expressed as a function of drug concentration, as for example that data given in figure 7. This shows that L8711 is a more efficient sensitizer than L9451 which is more efficient than Ro-07-0582 (misonidazole) i.e., a lower concentration is required to achieve the same biological response.

From data such as that in figure 7 it has been possible to correlate sensitizing efficiency with electron affinity for a wide range of different classes of nitro compounds[10, 11, 12]. The compounds of highest electron affinity, like L8711, being the most efficient sensitizers. However, it

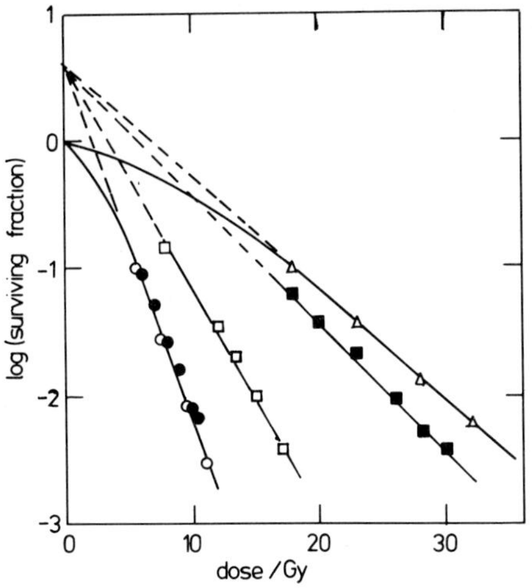

Fig. 6. Survival curves for V79-379A cells in the presence of several different radiosensitizers: △ , N_2 alone; ■ , N_2 + 0.2 mmol dm^{-3} RGW-611; □ , N_2 + 0.5 mmol. dm^{-3} RGW-609; ○ , aerated cells alone; ● , aerated cells with 0.5 mmol. dm^{-3} RGW-609.

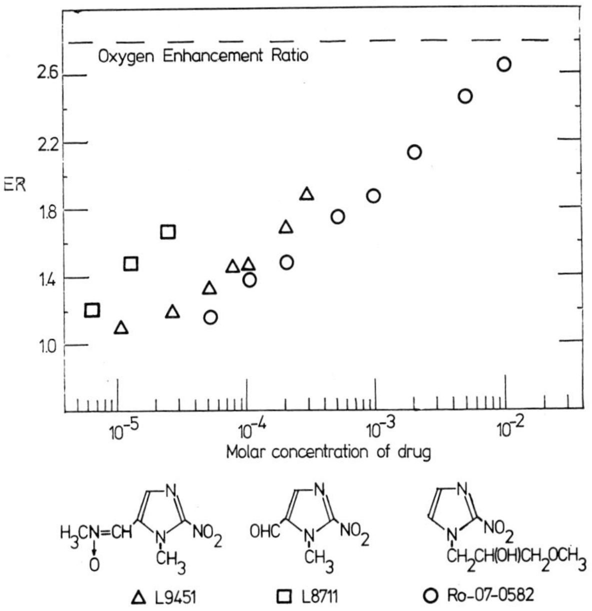

Fig. 7. The dependence of enhancement ratios of radiosensitization of hypoxic Chinese hamster V79-379A cells on drug concentration.

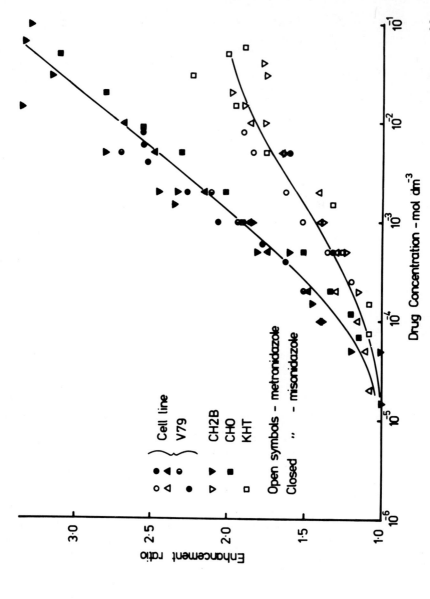

Fig. 8. The sensitization of a variety of cell lines by misonidazole and metronidazole. O , Asquith et al.[16]; ●, Asquith et al.[17]; ⊗, Chapman et al.[18]; ◉ , Hall and Roizin-Towle[19]; ▼ , Moore et al.[20]; ▽ Palcic[21]; ■ , Wong and Whitmore[22]; ▢ , Thomson and Rauth[23].

should be noted that L8711 and L9451 (figure 7) were not tested at higher
concentrations because they became toxic and it has been shown that the
aerobic toxicity of these compounds shows a similar dependence on red-ox
properties as does radiosensitization i.e., compounds of higher electron-
affinity are toxic at lower concentrations[13, 14]. This similarity in behaviour
should allow considerable manipulation of drug design to allow testing
in vivo of compounds that minimise the physiological responses that are
dose limiting in the clinical use of these compounds at the present
time (viz. for misonidazole and metronidazole neurotoxicity is the limiting
response).

4. FURTHER IN VITRO TESTING OF SENSITIZERS

4.1. Sensitization in a variety of cell lines

Figure 8 shows some of the published data on the sensitization by
misonidazole and metronidazole of various cells lines *in vitro*. The plot
of enhancement ratio versus drug concentration would appear to be relatively
independent of the cell line used. Indeed, a comparison has been made of
the sensitization seen in these *in vitro* cell lines with tumour responses,
when the concentration of misonidazole in the tumour was known at the time
of irradiation[15]. This showed that the sensitizer enhancement ratios achieved
in 4 different animals tumours correlated extremely well with what you would
expect from the *in vitro* data figure 8. This would lead us to predict that
any sensitizer will be active *in vivo* if it remains unmetabolized, can
penetrate to the hypoxic regions of tumours and be there at the time of
irradiation.

4.2. Sensitization with radiations of different quality

For the results presented so far X- and γ-rays have been used as the
type of radiations. These are low LET radiations. Clinically, in radiotherapy
treatment high LET radiation, such as neutrons or heavy particles, can also
be used and several groups have determined whether sensitizing efficiency
alters with these radiations[24,25,26,27]. Data in Table 1, obtained by
McNally[25], shows that for three different sensitizers the enhancement ratio
(ER) for each of the radiosensitizers decreases as the oxygen enhancement
ratio (OER) decreases.

TABLE 1

Compound	Radiation	OER	ER	ER/OER
5mM misonidazole	X-rays	2.72	2.26	0.73
(Ro-07-0582)	neutrons	1.65	1.57	0.88
0.4mM p nitro-	X-rays	2.98	1.71	0.36
acetophenone	neutrons	1.69	1.24	0.35
0.1mM nifurpipone	X-rays	2.96	1.70	0.36
	neutrons	1.74	1.33	0.45

These results support the suggestion that these nitroaromatic sensitizers act in a similar fashion to oxygen[28] with the amount of sensitization, as a proportion of the OER, independent of the quality of the radiation.

4.3. Studies with synchronized cells

The radiation sensitivity of cells varies throughout the cell cycle[29], with cells in S phase more resistant than those in other phases. For sensitizers to be most effective clinically it is essential that they are active throughout the cell cycle. Figure 9 shows some data for the sensitizers nitrofurazone, nitrofurantoin and misonidazole obtained with Chinese hamster V79 cells[8,17]. For each of these drugs sensitization occurs to the same extent throughout the cell cycle i.e., the amount of sensitization in S phase is the same as the amount of sensitization in G_1 etc. This finding is added evidence for these compounds acting in an O_2-mimetic fashion, since oxygen also increases radiation sensitivity equally throughout the cell cycle. Similar cell cycle studies have been carried out with misonidazole in NHIK cells, a cell line derived from a human uterine cervix carcinoma. This work confirmed the O_2-mimetic character of misonidazole[30,31].

4.4. Serum effects and protein binding studies

These studies are an extremely important part of sensitizer testing and evaluation. Any compound which is promising enough to go into *in vivo* testing must not be affected by serum protein. Generally, protein binding does not occur with the nitroimidazoles currently under investigation. However, at an earlier stage of sensitizer development the p-nitroacetophenone derivative NDPP was found to be not as effective *in vivo* as would have been anticipated from *in vitro* data[32]. The ability of this compound to act as a sensitizer is interfered with by serum protein.

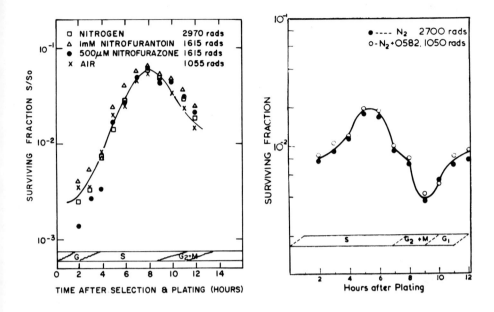

Fig. 9.   Radiosensitization of V79 cells at various stages of the cell cycle by nitrofurantoin, nitrofurazone and misonidazole (Ro 07-0582). Cells were synchronized with hydroxyurea.

In the evaluation of potential sensitizers radiation experiments are now carried out in medium containing varying concentrations of serum. If sensitization remains constant as a function of serum concentration then this is a good indication that, for subsequent *in vivo* studies, protein binding will not have any effect on the sensitizer response.

5. THE DIFFERENTIAL TOXIC EFFECT OF NITROAROMATIC RADIOSENSITIZERS

Sutherland in 1974[33] made the observation that the sensitizer metronidazole was specifically toxic to the non-cycling cells in the *in vitro* spheroid. Then, for misonidazole, the toxicity was found to be specifically directed at hypoxic cells[19]. This specific or differential toxicity towards hypoxic cells has subsequently been found to be associated with a whole range of electron-affinic nitroaromatic compounds, which also act as radiosensitizers[34].

Fig. 10 shows typical data illustrating the magnetude of this differential toxic effect at 37°C[35]. In this particular experiment cells were kept in contact with drug for varying periods of time under either hypoxic or fully

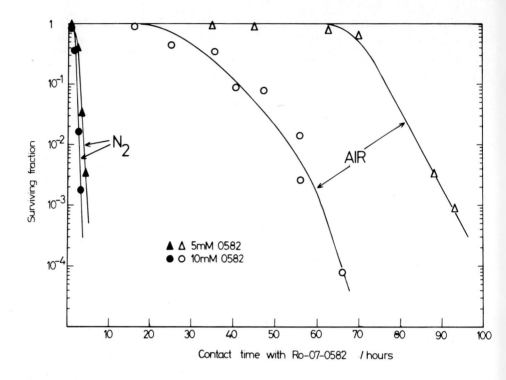

Fig. 10. The cytotoxic effect of misonidazole towards aerobic and hypoxic mammalian cells.

aerobic conditions. Clearly, cells in hypoxia are much more susceptable to killing by misonidazole than aerobic cells. The magnetude of the differential effect is best shown by comparing data for 5mM misonidazole, where under hypoxic conditions the surviving fraction of 10^{-3} is reached in 4 hours, in contrast, in air it takes 4 <u>days</u> to reduce survival to this level.

   The implication of these findings are considerable, for it may allow the eradication of hypoxic cells by chemotherapeutic action in addition to any radiosensitizing effect. This will be important in cancer chemotherapy where hypoxic cells may be a problem, since recent data from Smith, Stratford and Adams[36] has shown that some chemotherapeutic drugs in current use are less active towards hypoxic cells (previously growing exponentially) than compared to aerobic cells in log phase. Because of the potential importance of these observations it is practice now, in the evaluation of nitro compounds as radiosensitizers, to test their ability to act as

cytotoxic agents towards hypoxic cells. This is done by methods similar
to those described in section 2.1. for the radiation treatment of single
cell populations. The most convenient of these methods is that using cells
in suspension, where cells can be treated easily under any gaseous condition
or at various temperatures[37]. After the desired exposure time to the compound
under test samples of cell suspension can be removed and the number of surviving
cells assayed.

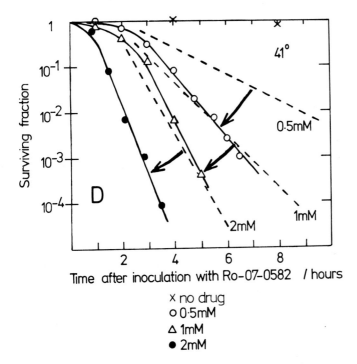

Fig. 11. The effect of increasing temperature on the hypoxic cell toxicity
of misonidazole toward V79-379A cells. Dashed lines, those survival curves
obtained at 37°C for 0.5, 1 and 2 mmol. dm^{-3} misonidazole. Solid lines
represent survival curves obtained at 41°C. X, no drug; O , 0.5 mmol.; $\triangle$ 1 mmol.
dm^{-3} misonidazole; ● , 2 mmol. dm^{-3} misonidazole.

The temperature at which these toxicity experiments are carried out
is very critical as is well illustrated in figure 11. Here, increasing
temperature from 37°C (dashed line) to 41°C (solid lines) produces a considerable
increase in toxicity, the 4° rise in temperature causing about a factor
of 2 increase in toxicity[37]. This result suggests that the application

of modest hyperthermia will increase any antitumour effect of these compounds. Decreasing the temperature below 37°C progressively decreases the toxicity, which is a likely reason why this differential toxic effect was found relatively late in radiosensitizer development, because initially all studies were carried out at room temperature. At ambient temperature the magnetude of the differential toxic effect becomes much smaller.

Hypoxic cell toxicity can also be modified by pH[38], which is illustrated in figure 12. Over the time course of these experiments pH _per se_ has no effect on cell survival under hypoxic conditions, but with misonidazole

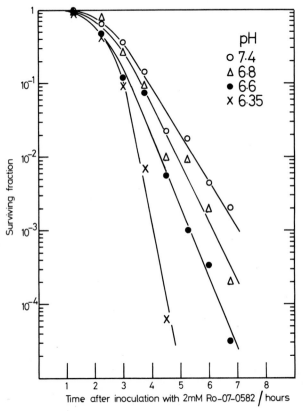

Fig. 12. The effect of varying pH on the toxicity of misonidazole towards hypoxic mammalian cells.

present toxicity is much greater at lower pH. For example, after 5 hours exposure at pH 6.35 survival is reduced to 10^{-5}, whereas at pH 7.4 the surviving fraction is only 10^{-2}.

The effect of temperature and pH clearly demonstrate a difference

between the mechanisms of drug cytotoxicity and the mechanisms of radiation
sensitization. These and some other differences, which have been noted for
mosonidazole are given in Table II. In addition, it appears that cytotoxicity
is dependent upon the presence of a nitro group in an aromatic nucleus of
high electron affinity, which is not the case for sensitization which can also
be seen with quinones [28] etc. At the present time there is good evidence to
suggest that radiation sensitization by oxygen and electron-affinic compounds
occurs via a fast free-radical mechanism[44], whereas cytotoxicity is a consequence of anaerobic metabolic reduction of the nitro group in these componds.

TABLE II

Treatment	Cytotoxicity	Sensitization
Temperature	Increasing toxicity with increasing temperature[37,39]	No effect
pH	Increasing toxicity with decreasing pH[38]	No effect
Cell line dependence	Magnetude of toxicity varies with cell line	Independent of cell line
Serum effect	Toxicity dependen on serum batch and concentration[47]	Generally independent of serum batch and concentration[12]
Hyperthermia/split dose experiments	No inhibition of split dose repair[42]	Split dose repair inhibited[43]
Timescale	Hours	1 s[44]

6. CONCLUSION

These data illustrate some of the principles and methods involved in the
development of nitro compounds as radiosensitizers and also as potential
cytotoxic agents. At the present time it is relatively easy to predict the
likely efficiency of any particular compounds as a radiosensitizer. The
limiting factor for future prospects is the development of an assay (in vitro
or in vivo) which will accurately reflect the possible neurotoxic effects of
a potential radiosensitizer. With such an advance the achievement of the best
hypoxic cell radiosensitizer might be a reality.

REFERENCES

1. Dawson, K.B., Madoc-Hones, H., Mauro, F. and Peacock, J.H., (1973) Eur. J. Cancer, 9, 59-68.

2. Barendsen, G.W. and Broerse, J.J., (1969) Eur. J. Cancer, 5, 373-391.

3. Chapman, J.D. and Boag, J.W., (1968) Br. J. Radiol., 41, 951-952.

4. Cooke, B.C., Fielden, E.M., Johnson, M. and Smithen, C.E., (1976) Radiat. Res., 65, 152-162.

5. Parker, L., Skarsgard, L.D. and Emmerson, P.T., (1969) Radiat. Res., 38, 493-500.

6. Hall, E.J., Lehnert, S. and Roizin-Towle, L., ($\frac{1}{2}$974) Radiology, 112, 425-430.

7. Sutherland, R.M. and Durand, R.E., (1976) Curr. Top. Radiat. Res. Quart., 11, 87-139.

8. Chapman, J.D., Reuvers, A.P., Borsa, J., Petkau, A. and McCalla, D.R., (1972) Cancer Res., 32, 2616-2624.

9. Wardman, P., (1977) Curr. Top. Radiat. Res. Quart., 11, 347-398.

10. Adams, G.E., Clarke, E.D., Flochart, I.R., Jacobs, R.S., Sehmi, D.S., Stratford, I.J., Wardman, P., Watts, M.E., Parrick, J., Wallace, R.G. and Smithen, C.E., (1978) Int. J. Radiat. Biol., (in press).

11. Rayliegh, J.A., Chapman, J.D., Borsa, J., Kramers, W. and Reuvers, A.P., (1973) Int. J. Radiat. Biol., 23, 377-387.

12. Adams, G.E., Flockhart, I.R., Smithen, C.E., Stratford, I.J., Wardman, P. and Watts, M.E., (1976) Radiat. Res., 67, 9-20.

13. Adams, G.E., Clarke, E.D., Jacobs, R.S., Stratford, I.J., Wallace, R.G., Wardman, P. and Watts, M.E., (1976) Biochem. Biophys. Res. Comm., 72, 824-829.

14. Adams, G.E., Clarke, E.D., Gray, P., Jacobs, R.S., Stratford, I.J., Wardman, P., Watts, M.E., Parrick, J., Wallace, R.G. and Smithen, C.E., (1978) Int. J. Radiat? Biol., (in press).

15. McNally, N.J., Denekamp, J., Sheldon, P., Flockhart, I.R. and Stewart, F.A., (1978) Rad. Res., 73, 568-580.

16. Asquith, J.C., Foster, J.L. and Willson, R.L., (1974) Br. J. Radiol.,

47, 474-481.

17. Asquith, J.C., Watts, M.E., Patch, K., Smithen, C.E. and Adams, G.E., (1974) Rad. Res., 6°, 108-118.

18. Chapman, J.D., Reuvers, A.P. and Borsa, J., (1973) Br. J. Radiol., 46, 623-63°.

19. Hall, E.J. and Roizin-Towle, L., (1975) Radiology, 117, 453-457.

20. Moore, B.A., Palcic, B. and Skarsgard, L.D., (1976) Rad. Res., 67, 459-473.

21. Palcic, B., (1974) Data presented at Radiosensitizer Workshop, Seattle, U.S.A., June 1974.

22. Wong, T.W. and Whitmore, G.F., (1977) Rad. Res., 71, 132-148.

23. Thomson, J.E. and Rauth, A.M., (1974) Rad. Res., 6°, 489-500.

24. Hall, E.J., Roizin-Towle, L., Theus, R.B. and August, L.S., (1975) Radiology, 117, 173-179.

25. McNally, N.J., (1976) Int. J. Radiat. Biol., 29, 191-196.

26. Chapman, J.D., Urtason, R.C., Blakely, E.A., Smith, K.C. and Tobias, C.A., (1978) Br. J. Cancer, 37, Suppl III, 184-188.

27. Raju, M.R., Amols, H.J. and Carpenter, S.G., (1978) Br. J. Cancer, 37, Suppl III, 189-193.

28. Adams, G.E. and Cooke, M.S., (1969) Int. J. Radiat. Biol., 15, 457-471.

29. Terasima, T. and Tolmach, L.J., (1963) Biophys. J., 3, 11-33.

30. Pattersen, E.O., Christense, T., Bakke, O. and Oftebro, R., (1977) Int. J. Radiat. Biol., 31, 171-184.

31. Pattersen, E.O., (1978) Rad. Res., 180-191.

32. Rauth, A.M., Kaufman, K. and Thomson, J.E., (1975) in Radiation Research-Biomedical, Chemical and Physical Perspectives, Nygaars, O.F., Adler, H.I. and Sinclair, W.K. eds., Academic Press, New York, pp. 761-772.

33. Sutherland, R.M., (1974) Cancer Res., 34, 3501-3503.

34. Adams, G.E., Stratford, I.J., Wardman, P. and Watts, M.E., (1978) J. Natl. Cancer Inst., (submitted for publication).

35. Stratford, I.J., WATTS, M.E. and Adams, G.E., ($\frac{1}{2}$978) in Cancer Therapy by Hyperthermia and Radiation, Streffer, C. ed., Urban and Schwarzenberg, Baltimore-Munich, pp. 267-270.

36. Smith, E., Stratford, I.J. and Adams, G.E., (1978) manuscript in preparation.

37. Stratford, I.J. and Adams, G.E., (1977) Br. J. Cancer, 35, 3°7-313.

38. Stratford, I.J., (1977) Int. J. Radiat. Biol., 32, 279.

39. Hall, E.J., Astor, M., Geard, C. and Biaglow, J., (1977) Br. J. Cancer, 35, 809-815.

40. Taylor, Y.C. and Rauth, A.M., (1978) Cancer Res., 38, 2745-2752.

41. Stratford, I.J. and Gray, P., (1978) Br. J. Cancer, 37, Suppl III, 129-131.

42. Stratford, I.J., (1978) Br. J. Cancer, 38, 130-136.

43 Ben-Hur, E., Elkind, M.M. and Bronk, B.V., (1974) Rad. Res., 58, 38-51.

44. Adams, G.E., Michael, B.D., Asquith, J.C., Shenoy, M.A., Watts, M.E., and Whillans, D.W., (1975) in Radiation Research-Biomedical, Chemical and Physical Perspectives, Nygaard, O.F., Adler, H.I. and Sinclair, W.K. eds., Academic Press, New York, pp. 478-492.

IN VIVO RADIOSENSITIZATION: PRINCIPLES AND METHODS OF STUDY

JACK F. FOWLER

Gray Laboratory of Cancer Research Campaign, Mount Vernon Hospital, Northwood, Middlesex, HA6 2RN, England.

ABSTRACT

The role of animal experiments in helping to develop the clinical applications of hypoxic cell radiosensitizers can be described under four headings;

1) To compare the potential advantages of radiosensitizers with those of other treatments, in the same tumour and normal-tissue systems.

2) To compare the disadvantageous side-effects with the advantageous effects on tumours.

3) To find optimum ways of using the radiosensitizers: the "best scheduling".

4) To help in the design and testing of new radiosensitizers.

Details of the various methods of measuring the response of experimental tumours in mice or rats are presented, together with results.

TUMOUR RESPONSE TO SINGLE DOSES OF HYPOXIC-CELL RADIOSENSITIZER

We do not rely on results from only one experimental tumour system. We use at least four and preferably six types of mouse tumour with any new modality and look for differences in response. It is only if a very general effect is found, as here, that we can feel confident that the method is likely to be reliable in a variety of human tumours. The mouse tumour results were in fact less variable for misonidazole than they have been for hyperbaric oxygen, or neutrons, or hyperthermia (Tables 1, 2)[1]. This constant finding has helped the ready acceptance of clinicians to embark on clinical trials using hypoxic cell radiosensitizers. The other factor which has led to clinical acceptance in the good co-operation at Mount Vernon Hospital between the Gray Laboratory and the clinicians. Dr. Dische had establisched clinically that the limiting dose of misonidazole was $12g/m^2$ to avoid the neurotoxic side effects, by the

TABLE 1

RADIOSENSITIZATION TO SINGLE DOSES OF X-RAYS BY MISONIDAZOLE (Ro-07-0582)

Tumour	Assay System	Sensitizer Enhancement Ratio for drug dose administered (mg/g)				Interval between admin. & irrad. (mins)	Reference
		0.1	0.2-0.3	0.5-0.7	1.0-1.5		
C3H MICE							
Mam. Ca	Local control	-	1.7-1.8	-	1.8	30	Sheldon et al., 74
Mam. Ca	"	-	-	-	2.3	30	Stone & Withers, 75b
Mam. Ca	"	-	1.8	-	2.3	30	Brown, 75
Fibro Sa	"	-	-	-	1.6	30	Stone (pers. commun.)
Sa KHT	Excision and lung colonies	-	-	-	1.9	60	Rauth et al., 75
CBA MICE							
Ca NT	Regrowth delay	1.5	1.9	2.1	2.2.	15-25	Denekamp & Harris, 75 & unpublished
Sa F	"	-	-	-	2.0	30	McNally, 75.
Sa F	"	-	-	-	1.7	30	Begg, 77
Sa F	^{125}IUdR loss.	-	~1.0	~1.0	1.5	30	"
Sa F	Excision in vitro surv.	-	1.3	-	2.2	30	McNally, 75
Slow SaS	Regrowth delay	-	-	-	~1.0	15-20	Denekamp et al., 78
Discoid Ca	"	-	-	-	1.6	15-20	" " "
Sa FFl	"	-	-	-	1.7	15-20	" " "

TABLE I - Continued

BALB/C MICE

EMT 6	Excision/in vitro surv.	2.4	2.7	2.4	2.9	30-45	Brown, 75

WHT/Ht MICE

Sq. Ca G	Local control	-	1.9	-	2.0	20-30	Peters, 76
Sq. Ca D	"	-	-	-	2.0	30	Hill & Fowler, 77
Sq. Ca D	Regrowth delay	-	-	-	2.2.	30	"
Anaplast.MT	"	-	-	-	1.8	30	Sheldon & Hill, 77
Anaplast.MT	Local control	1.5	1.6-1.7	-	2.1	30	"
Anaplast.MT	Excision/in vitro surv.	-	-	-	1.6	30	McNally & Sheldon, 77
Rhod. Ca	Regrowth delay	1.4	-	-	1.4	15-20	Denekamp et al., 78
Bone Sa 2	"	-	-	1.7	1.8	15-30	"
Fibro Sa	"	-	-	1.9	1.9	15-20	"

RAT

Sa 180	^{125}IUdR loss	-	-	1.5	-	15-90	Porschen et al., 77

ARTIFICIALLY HYPOXIC SKIN

		1.4	1.6	-	2.2	10-20	Denekamp et al., 74

*Significant radiosensitization has been observed in all experimental tumours except Sa F at low drug doses because of the insensitivity of the ^{125}IUdR assay (Begg, 77), and in the slow sarcoma S where no hypoxic cells are present.

TABLE 2

RADIOSENSITIZATION TO SINGLE DOSES OF X-RAYS BY METRONIDAZOLE (FLAGYL)

Tumour	Assay System	Sensitizer enhancement ratio for drug dose administered (mg/g):						Interval between admin. & irrad. (mins)	Reference
		0.1	0.25	0.75	1.0	1.5	2.5		
C3H Mam	Local control	-	-	-	-	-	1.4	30	Begg et al., 74
"	"	1.2	-	-	-	-	-	30	Stone & Withers, 74, 75a
CBA Sa F	125JUdR loss	-	-	-	1.5	1.6	-	30	Begg et al., 74
"	Regrowth delay	-	-	-	-	1.6	-	30	"
CBA Ca NT	"	-	-	1.6	-	-	-	20-30	Denekamp & Harris, 75
C3H Sa KHT	Excision & lung colonies	-	-	-	-	1.5	-	15	Rauth & Kaufman, 75
EMT 6	Excision & in vitro surviv.	-	-	-	1.8	-	-	30	Brown, 75
WHT Sq	Local control	-	1.3	-	-	-	-	20-30	Peters, 76
WHT MT	"	1.2	-	-	1.5	-	-	30	Sheldon & Hill, 77
ARTIFICIALLY HYPOXIC SKIN		1.2	1.2	-	1.3	1.3	1.3-1.5	10-20	Denekamp et al., 74

These enhancement ratios have been derived from pairs of dose response curves where the dose needed to produce the same level of damage in the presence and absence of the drug has been determined.

time that many of the mouse tumour results had become published and known
about.

In our laboratory we use only tumours which arose spontaneously in mice
of three inbred strains. Each type of tumour is transplanted only in its strain
of origin. The tumours are therefore free of the immune reactivity which is
found in tumours induced by strong carcinogenic chemicals or viruses, or in
tumours transplanted into animals other than the strain of origin. Results
of our experiments cannot be interpreted as merely artefacts of boosting the
immune response of the animals to their experimental tumours.

The single-dose experiments in Tables 1 and 2 show one tumour only with
no enhancement for misonidazole at high dose. This is a slow-growing sarcoma
which has few or no hypoxic cells[2]. It is only in slow-growing sarcomas that
the absence of cell loss is likely to lead to no hypoxic cells. Carcinomas
are likely to contain hypoxic cells even if they are slow-growing[3].

METHODS OF STYDYING TUMOUR RESPONSE

a) Regrowth Delay[4]

This well-known method can be used with any type of tumour that grows as
a solid lump, without diffuse edges, and which does not kill the animal by
metastases within about a month. The results are obtained about a month after
irradiation, sometimes longer for very slow-growing tumours. A major advantage
is that a wide range of radiation doses can be used, from a few hundred rads
to several kilorads and all dose groups will provide data. Eight to ten mice
are required per dose point. No discrepancies have been found between this
and the following method, although the volume of the tumour is not simply
proportional to the number of viable cells in it.

b) Local Control[5]

This method is even more obvious than regrowth delay. It cannot however
be used with as many types of tumour because the results take longer to obtain
so that metastases are more likely to kill the animals first. Another
disadvantage is that the proportion of tumours locally controlled (i.e. mice
cured) rises from 0 to 100% in a relatively narrow dose range. Dose groups
outside this range will contribute no useful data. Ten to twenty animals are

134

required per dose group. The results are obtained at the earliest in about 2½ months (for a tumour with a doubling time as short as one day) and often in 5 or 6 months. The precision of determination of the resulting dose required to control 50% of the tumours, the TCD_{50}, is good. Standard errors less than 5% are often recorded[6]. Figure 1 shows single-dose results for misonidazole using this method. The shaded area represents the improvement of results obtained for tumour concentrations in the clinical range. A larger dose of misonidazole per unit body weight has to be given to mice than to man because

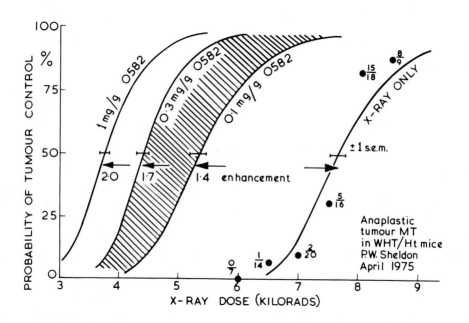

Fig. 1. Probability of tumor control (i.e; mouse cure) at 80 days for the anaplastic MT tumor in WHT mice. The X-rays only TCD_{50} was halved when 1mg/g of misonidazole was injected i.p. 30 mins before irradiation. The shaded area represents the concentration range in the tumors that is obtenable in patients.

the short half-life in mice results in no more than 30-50% of the serum
concentration appearing in the tumour, whereas in man it is usually 60-100%.
This range of sensitizer enhancement ratios* is 1.4 to 1.7 for misonidazole.
It overlaps the range of therapeutic gain factors obtained with fast neutrons,
which is 1.6 to 1.8.

c) Excision of Tumours and Testing in Vitro or in Vivo

After certain types of experimental tumour have been treated in vivo, they
can be cut out, and the cells dispersed into a single-cell suspension. The
proportion of these cells which survived the treatment can then be counted
in vitro by growing the cells in culture for 1 to 3 weeks[7]; or in vivo by
injecting into other test mice to see how many tumour cells are viable. For
example, cell survival curves can be obtained by injecting cell suspensions
into the tail vein of mice and counting the number of colonies growing in the
lungs 2 or 3 weeks later[8]. Alternatively, successively diluted cell suspensions
can be injected subcutaneously into several sites in each mouse, and the later
growth of tumours recorded[9]. This method yields the "TD_{50}", the "50% Take Dose",
which is the number of injected cells required to produce a tumour in 50% of
the test sites. It must be distinguished from the TCD_{50} described above.

The excision method is the quickest and most economical of mice but has
several disadvantages. Results can be obtained in 2 to 3 weeks and only 2
or 3 mice per dose point are needed. However not many types of tumour can be
dispersed into single-cell suspensions. A serious problem arises in some
tumours because of the repair of "potentially lethal damage", PLD. Each
tumour in which this test is to be used has to be validated for the absence
of repair of PLD. The time between irradiation and excision has to be varied
from 0 up to 16 or more hours (when proliferation would begin and would be
another invalidating factor). If the resulting number of surviving cells is
the same for any time interval the method is valid. In some tumours, however,
the proportion of cells which survive irradiation increases with time. In

---

*Sensitizer Enhancement Ratio (SER) is defined as the ratio of

X-ray dose without sensitizer
X-ray dose with sensitizer

required to produce a stated biological effect.

such tumours the assay can only be done when the number has become constant, i.e. when repair of the PLD is complete. This procedure should give the nearest match to in situ tests described above. However, divergences between the in situ tests and the excision methods have often been reported. Thus although the excision methods are quick, economical, and yield cell survival curves, the results may be less relevant to what happens in a tumour left in situ than results from the regrowth delay or tumour control methods.

d) Loss of Cells Labelled with ^{125}IUdR

All the cells in a mouse that are synthesizing DNA in preparation for cell division can be labelled by a "flash label", a single injection of a precursor of DNA. Iodo-desoxyuridine labelled with radioactive iodine-125 is used, a few microcuries being given intraperitoneally. Twenty-four or forty-eight hours later, to allow ^{125}I not bound into DNA to be removed, the mouse can be anaesthetised and its tumour counted in part of a collimated radiation detector. The percentage of ^{125}I remaining in the tumour is plotted against time. It is a rough measure of how many cells remain in the tumour, because radioactivity can only be lost from the DNA when the cell is destroyed. The percentage of ^{125}I falls gradually for 7 to 10 days in untreated (control) tumours but more rapidly if the tumour has been treated. The effect of 1000 rads of x-rays alone can be distinguished from that of 500 or 1500 rads. If giving misonidazole to the mice before irradiation results in the 500 rad curve becoming as steep as that for 1000 rads with x-rays only, an SER of 2.0 would be indicated[10]. This method has the advantage of being quick, 7 or 10 days, but it requires 8-10 mice per dose group and can only be used after each type of tumour has been well investigated to "calibrate" its rate of loss of radioactivity[11]. The method cannot be used for x-rays doses above about 2000 rads because the loss rate does not increase further. Some tumours contain the artifact of "reutilization", where during the first one or two days they may take up more radioactivity, from other cells in the body which lose it, than they lose. This can be corrected for in the preliminary calibration but is in principle undesirable.

COMPARISON BETWEEN IN VIVO AND IN VITRO SER's

The methods described in the previous section were used to obtain the results listed in Tables 1 and 2. Dose of drug per unit bodyweight is an unsatisfactory measure however. McNally et al[12] have recently found that the SER values are similar for four types of mouse tumour in vivo to those of hamster V79 cells in vitro, when plotted against the measured concentration of radiosensitizer in the tumour or in the culture medium (Fig. 2). They are

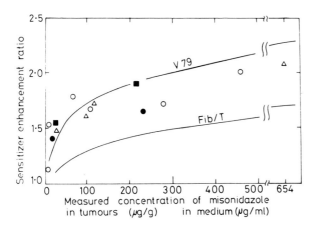

Fig. 2. Enhancement ratios plotted as a function of the measured drug concentration in the tumour at the time of irradiation. The upper line is for V79 379A Chinese hamster cells *in vitro*, and the lower one is for Fib/T cells *in vitro*.
○ Fib/T; △ MT; ■ NT¹; ● BS2.

higher than the values for a line of malignant cells in culture (lower curve). At the low concentrations relevant to human tumours (20-100µg/ml) the SER values were somewhat higher in vivo than in vitro. There is certainly no "loss factor" in vivo, provided that the tumour concentrations are known reliably.

MISONIDAZOLE AND FAST NEUTRONS

The single-dose SER for misonidazole varies from 1.7 to over 2.0 for large doses of 1mg/g body weight. In the C3H mouse tumour it was 1.7, which was the same as the hypoxic gain factor[*] obtained with cyclotron neutrons. The improvement of tumour results for misonidazole was the same as for neutrons, both for single doses and multiple fractions. This point is explained in more detail in my other paper in this Course, and in the following section.

MULTIPLE FRACTION SCHEDULES WITH MISONIDAZOLE

Table 3 shows that the SER's are smaller for multiple fractions than for single doses. This occurs for two reasons. First, if reoxygenation occurs during the treatment schedule, there will be fewer hypoxic cells as a problem, and the maximum SER required to eliminate them all will be less. Second, smaller individual doses of radiosensitizer are obviously given as multiple fractions

TABLE 3

SENSITIZER ENHANCEMENT RATIOS FOR FRACTIONATED IRRADIATIONS

Tumour	Drug dose per fraction (mg/g)	Single dose	2F	3F	5F	Reference
MISONIDAZOLE						
CBA Ca NT	0.67	2.1	1.6	-	1.3	Denekamp and Harris, 76b
C3H Ca Mam.	0.67-1.0	1.8	-	1.1	1.2	Fowler et al., 76
	0.67 (5F/4d)				1.1	Sheldon et al., 75
WHT MT	0.33	1.7	-	-	1.5	Sheldon et al., 77
	Any 2 out of 5F	-	-	-	1.3	" " "
WHT Bone Sa 2	0.67	1.7	1.5	-	-	Denekamp et al., 78
WHT Fibro Sa	0.67	1.9	-	-	1.1	" "
METRONIDAZOLE						
C3H Ca Mam.	0.1	1.2	-	-	1.1	Stone, 76
(MDAH-MCa-4)	1.0	1.5	-	-	1.3	"

The SER decreases with longer fractionation. It is due, in some tumours, to loss of effectiveness of the radiosensitizer as reoxygenation proceeds. In others it is merely a reflection of the fact that sensitization equivalent to (say) 1000 rads is a large proportion of a single dose but a smaller proportion of the fractionated total dose.

---

[*]Hypoxic gain factor for neutrons = OER for x-rays divided by OER for neutrons

than as single doses. It should be noted that a similar drop in gain factor occurs with neutrons on changing from one to several fractions. However, such a drop in the dose ratios does not necessarily mean that the proportion of tumours cured will be less, as illustrated in Fig. 3. On the left an SER of

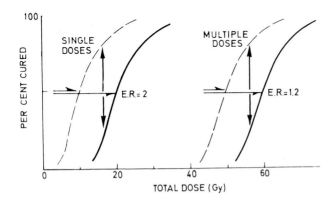

Fig. 3. A single dose SER of 2 and a fractionated SER of 1.2 both give the same improvment in cure.

2.0 is shown: 50% local control for 2000 rads of x-rays only or 1000 rads of x-rays with sensitizer. The difference is 1000 rads and the consequent increase of effect is from, say, 30% to 60%. On the right of Fig. 3 is the same increase of effect, with the same difference of 1000 rads, for a multi-fraction schedule. Hare the doses are 6000 rads without, and 5000 rads with, the sensitizer; so the SER is only 1.2. This is large enough to be clinically detectable with only 200 or 300 patients, but smaller values of SER would be impractical to demonstrate.

A large series of experiments was carried out with our first-generation C3H mouse mammary tumours transplanted into the same strain of mice[13]. About a dozen different fractionation schedules were employed, and a dose-response curve for tumour control was determined for each schedule. Skin reaction dose-response curves were obtained in other mice for the same schedules. It was then possible to find the dose required in a given schedule to yield an average skin reaction of 2.0 (severe desquamation which healed in 6 weeks) and to look up, on the tumour response curve for that schedule, what proportion of tumours were locally controlled by that dose.

Fig. 4 shows these results for x-rays only, all for the same degree of normal tissue damage to skin of mice. The volume doubling times of the tumours were 4-6 days so "days" in fig. 4 might be considered as "weeks" in human tumours, assuming volume doubling time is a valid scaling factor.

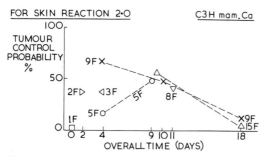

Fig. 4. X-rays only; several schedules.

It can be seen from Fig. 4 that when the treatment was given in too long an overall time - more than 11 days - the results were poor. The tumours had grown faster than the rate of cell killing. At the medium overall time of 9 or 10 days, all the results were equally good and the detailed fractionation did not matter. It was a kind of "optimum overall time" for this tumour. At shorter overall times the results were very variable, due to insufficient reoxygenation. It was known that 48 hour intervals enabled more reoxygenation to occur than 24 hour intervals, so 3F/4d was better than 5F/4d. Also 5F/9d was better still, because the longer overall time allowed more reoxygenation.

Fig. 5 shows the results of giving misonidazole before irradiation in some of the schedules[13a]. The single doses were improved from 0% to 65% and all the other schedules with sensitizers were also brought up to the same good level of 50-70%.

In fact, for the same degree of skin reaction, there were no longer any bad results at the short overall times. It begins to look as though shorter overall times would be better, if it were not for the problem of hypoxic cells in conventional radiotherapy. One of the major contribution that hypoxic-cell radiosensitizers could make would be to enable shorter overall

times than 5 or 6 weeks to be used reliably. The economic consequences of
the saving of time for patients, beds, staff, and radiotherapy equipment,
are obvious.

Neutrons may achieve a similar result to those described above for
misonidazole, as shown in Figs. 6 and 7 of my other paper in this Course.

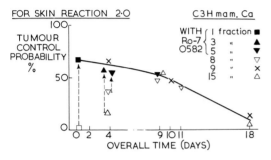

Fig. 5. Improvement in tumor control with misonidazole (vertical arrows).

ANIMAL EXPERIMENTS ON NORMAL TISSUES USING HYPOXIC-CELL RADIOSENSITIZERS

No radiosensitization of normal tissues has been seen except where it is
well known that a proportion of the cells were hypoxic. Denekamp, Harris and
Michael[14] have made skin deliberately hypoxic in order to measure the SER
values in vivo of various radiosensitizers being developed. A small proportion
of skin cells are hypoxic when mice are irradiated normally in air, so that
Foster[15] found a small SER for large single doses of X-rays with misonidazole
but no significant radiosensitization for 2 or 5 fractions. Hendry[16] has
found radiosensitization in the cartilage of mouse tails, which is indeed
normally hypoxic. He points out that there will be less radiosensitization
of normal tissues which are hypoxic in patients than in the case of hyperbaric
oxygen, where the effective OER was about 1.1. It is expected to be a smaller
problem than in HBO. Clinical results have so far not shown any enhancement
of normal tissue reactions at all (Dische, this Course). Nevertheless, few
animal experiments have been done to test this expectedly small problem and
more should be undertaken for completeness.

TESTING FOR SIDE EFFECTS

Toxicity testing for side effects has to be done in large animals before
a new drug can be used in man. Because this testing is expensive, some
selection of new compounds is necessary before the large-animal testing
will be started. With hypoxic-cell radiosensitizers, the sensitizing ability
can be predicted theoretically and measured reliably using mammalian cells in
vitro. It is not necessary to use mouse tumour systems to screen potential
new compounds, although some confirmation that a proposed drug will work in
vivo is necessary, as discussed in the final section.

Improved ways of assessing neurotoxicity in mice would be an advantage,
but we cannot be sure that all future radiosensitizers will have only than
as the main side effect. The main existing methods for toxicity testing in
mice or rats are traditional histology and pathology; and the rotating rod
off which they fall when their co-ordination weakens. Other methods are
experimental, such as the measurement of nerve conduction velocity in mice[17].

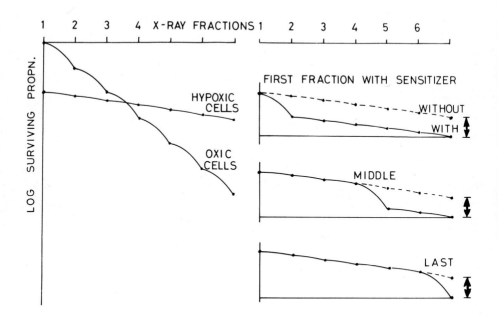

Fig. 6. Decrease in number of hypoxic cells as fractionated treatment proceeds.

The testing for toxic side effects is, at present, the slowest phase in the chain of development of new hypoxic-cell radiosensitizers.

SENSITIZER FIRST OR LAST?

If the use of a hypoxic-cell sensitizer is limited, by toxicity, to only a few of the many doses in a fractionated schedule, should they be the first ones, the last, or distributed throughout? The answer is the first ones, by a short lead. Although it makes no difference to the number of *hypoxic* cells remaining after treatment whether the sensitizer is given early or late (Fig.6), it does matter whenever *reoxygenation* is involved. Hypoxic cells should be reduced in number as quickly as possible, because their reoxygenation contributes most of the oxygenated cells in a tumour, after a few fractions. If hypoxic-cell sensitizers are used at the end of treatment, they have less effect (Fig. 7). Therefore there are fewer total cells remaining in the whole

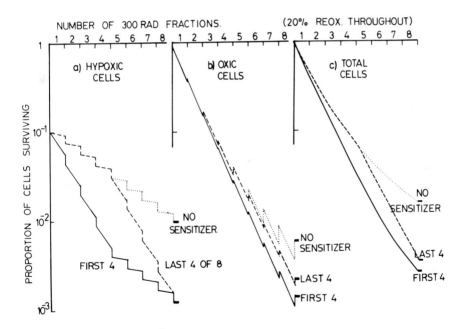

Fig. 7. Decrease in number of cells with repeated 300 rad fractions.

tumour if hypoxic-cell sensitizers are used at the beginning, not the end, of a schedule. The only exception to this would be if the *number* (not proportion) of hypoxic cells were increasing throughout the fractionated schedule, i.e. if the tumour continued to grow during treatment.

LARGE OR SMALL DOSES PER FRACTION?

This is a much-discussed question in the design of clinical trials. It is true that a few large doses, of radiation plus the drug, will enable a large SER to be obtained. Fig. 2 shows that an SER of about 1.6 is obtained for 70µg/ml, which is expected in tumours if six doses of 2mg/m^2 are used. Six times an SER of 1.6 is 1.6, so this enhancement will be achieved on hypoxic cells. If, however, 20 fractions of 0.6g/m^2 are used, the SER for each is about 1.3 and the combined SER will be 1.3 for the hypoxic cells.

It was shown in Fig. 3 that a lower SER for multiple fractions can give just as good a result as a higher one for a single dose. Further, Fig. 5 shows that a high SER for small numbers of fractions may lead to no better result than a low SER for multiple doses. There is no point in choosing a poor x-rays-only schedule deliberately to demonstrate "an effect". It would be better to schoose a good x-ray schedule, including multiple small daily fractions, and see whether that can be improved. The only limitation on subdividing doses is that if each drug dose gave a tumour concentration too low to expect an SER of at least 1.2 then the improvement, however real, would be too small to be detected in a clinical trial. However, the use of as many as 20 or 25 doses of 0.5-0.6g/m^2 misonidazole still enables 15-25µg/ml to be obtained in human tumours so that SER's above 1.2 are expected. Further subdivision, however, would lead to no detectable improvement. If the direct cytotoxicity to hypoxic cells is important, it is better to give a series of small daily doses than a few large ones.

The question of whether twice the drug dose should be given on alternate days has been raised. From the shape of the curve of SER versus drug concentration shown in Fig. 2, this is a disadvantage. Doubling the drug dose gives less than double the increment of SER above 1.0. If half the x-ray doses in a schedule are given with a sensitizer and half without, the resulting SER is the average of 1.0 and the SER with the sensitizer. If double the drug dose is given on alternate days, the SER will therefore be *less* than that obtained from using the sensitizer daily.

The size of *sensitizer dose per fraction* is important, and concentration in the tumour can be used in estimates of the maximum effect. However, this calculated SER may not be achieved fully if reoxygenation occurs. In this case, there would be no problem of hypoxic cells and the result should be as good as it can be, using x-rays. Sensitizers would help to ensure that this is so and that no hypoxic cells ramin unreoxygenated. This is important because we do not know in which human tumours reoxygenation is inadequate.

The size of radiation *dose per fraction* is of secondary importance. For a small dose of x-rays, the SER is of course reduced below the full value by the presence of oxic cells. This reduction will however change with time through a fractionated schedule, depending entirely on how effective reoxygenation is. If reoxygenation is poor, the SER for each dose fraction will increase to the full value. If reoxygenation is good, hypoxic cells will not be a problem anyway. Schedules with small doses per fraction are therefore entirely reasonable to use. Indeed, the significant improvement in the MRC hyperbaric oxygen trials when 25-27 fractions of 200 rads were used confirms this.

CYTOTOXIC EFFECT ON HYPOXIC CELLS

Table 4 shows that a significan cytotoxic effect (sensitizer given *after* irradiation) was seen in seven out of the fourteen types of tumour tested[19]. This is more than might have been expected, bearing in mind the short half-life of misonidazole in mice (1-1½ hours) and the long period of time (several hours) before cytotoxic cell killing becomes effective at 37°C. Most of these tumours in mice were at a lower temperature than body temperature, being at 33-35°C instead. Table IV suggests that an even larger contribution from direct cytotoxicity might be expected in human tumours (half life 10-15 hours). However, one word of caution is necessary. A small amount of reoxygenation, or cyclic oxygenation, in tumours will extend the time required for toxicity enormously. There is obviously more time for this to occur in human tumours

TABLE 4

CYTOTOXICITY AND RADIOSENSITIZATION: SUMMARY OF MOUSE TUMOURS.

ENHANCEMENT RATIOS OF 1 MG/G/MISONIDAZOLE IS GIVEN BEFORE OR AFTER IRRADIATION

After	Before	Tumour	Reference	After	Before	Tumour	Reference
1.2	2.3	C3H Ca	Brown, 1975	0.9	2.1	MT/1MT	Sheldon and Hill, 1977
1.3	2.2	Sq Ca D	Hill and Fowler, 1977	1.0	2.1	Fib/T	McNally (unpub.)
1.3	2.1	Ca NT	Denenkamp and Harris, 1975	1.0	1.8	B Sa 2	Denekamp (unpub.)
1.1	1.9	Fibrosa	Stewart (unpub.)	1.0	1.8	C3H Ca	Sheldon *et al.*, 1974
1.4	1.9	Rhod Ca	Denekamp (unpub.)	1.0	1.7	Disc Ca	Hirst (unpub.)
1.3	1.7	Sa F	Begg (unpub.)	1.0	1.7	FF Sa 1	Hirst (unpub.)
1.2	1.6	FFSa2	Hirst (unpub.)	1.0	1.5	Sa F	Begg (unpub.)
			7/14 Some cytotoxicity				7/14 No cytotoxicity

Drug given before irradiation demonstrates both cytotoxicity and radiosensitization

Drug given after irradiation demonstrates only cytotoxicity

than in the mouse tumours and, if it did, the effects in human tumours would be no greater than those in Table 4. If this cytotoxicity to hypoxic cells is important, many small fractions would be better than a few large ones.

ANIMAL EXPERIMENTS TO HELP IN THE DESIGN AND TESTING OF NEW RADIOSENSITIZERS

Whilst it is always satisfactory to confirm that a high SER measured in vitro can indeed be obtained in vivo, when the same concentration is measured in the tumour as was present in the culture medium, this will be a secondary finding if the result is satisfactory. Only if a discrepancy was found would it become of prime importance.

The first help that animal experiments can give in investigating a new drug is to detect extremely fast metabolism or extreme toxicity in vivo. Even then, these effects need to be tested on larger animals (with slower metabolism than mice) before a good radiosensitizer shoud be rejected from further studies.

It will always be useful to obtain relative concentrations of drug in serum and in experimental tumours, at different times after administration. In this way we shall be able to see how differences of lipophilicity or of charge on the sensitizer molecule affect the pharmacokinetics of drug uptake.

CONCLUSION

As Professor Adams and Dr. Wardman have explained in the present Course, the design and development of new radiosensitizers can be done rather precisely as regards the electron affinity, i.e. the radiosensitizing ability. This precision is a big advantage over other types of anti-cancer drug. The toxicity and pharmacology cannot yet be so well predicted however.

One of the most useful roles of animal experiments in the development of new drugs will be to test various ranges of "extreme" synthetic molecule, so as to gain insight into the molecular structural changes associated with toxicity in vivo. This is quite a difference strategy from the role of "picking the winner" from a group of new drugs presented for screening. It should, however, result in a much more logical, and eventually more certain, achievement of a worthy successor to misonidazole.

Animal experiments can then help to compare it to the best that can be done using neutrons, hyperthermia or combinations of x-rays with chemotherapy.

ACKNOWLEDGEMENTS

It is a pleasure to thank Professor Adams, Drs Denekamp, McNally, Wardman, Mr. Sheldon and others for stimulating discussions and for allowing me to quote their data as referred to. I thank the Editors of Brit. J. Cancer for permission to reproduce Figs. 1, 6 and 7; Brit. J. Radiol. for. Fig. 2; IAEA for Fig. 3; and Pergamon Press for Fig. 5.

REFERENCES

1. Fowler, J.F. and Kenekamp, J. (1978) A review of hypoxic cell radiosentization in experimental tumours. Pharmacology and Therapeutics (in press).

2. Reference 1, Table 4, Slow Sarcoma S. (also Denekamp, J. and Stewart, F.A., pers. comm.)

3. Denekamp, J. and Fowler, J.F. (1977) Cell proliferation kinetics and radiation therapy. Chapter 4 in "Cancer: a comprehensive treatise" Vol. 6, F.F. Becker ed., Plenum Press., pp. 101-137.

4. Denekamp, J. and Harris, S.R. (1975) Tests of two electron-affinic radio-sensitizers in vivo using regrowth of an experimental carcinoma. Radiat. Res., 61, 191-203.

5. Sheldon, P.W., Foster, J.L. and Fowler, J.F. (1974) Radiosensitization of C3H mouse mammary tumours by a 2-nitroimidazole drug. Brit. J. Cancer, 30, 560-565.

6. Sheldon, P.W. and Hill, S.A., (1977) Hypoxic cell radiosensitizers and local control by X-rays of a transplanted tumour in mice. Brit. J. Cancer, 35, 795-808.

7. McNally, N.J. (1972) Recovery from sublethal damage by hypoxic tumour cells in vivo, Br. J. Radiol., 45, 116-120.

8. Rauth, A.M. and Kaufman, K. (1975) In vivo testing of hypoxic radio-sensitizers using the KHT murine assayed by the lung colony technique. Brit. J. Radiol., 48, 209-220.

9. Hewitt, H.B. and Wilson, C.W. (1959) A survival curve for mammalian leukaemia cells in vivo. Brit. J. Cancer, 13, 69-75.

10. Porschen, W. and Feinendegen, L.E. (1973) Biologische in-vivo Dosimetrie von 15 MeV-Neutronen bei normalen und Tumorzellen wahrend des Zellzyklus, Zellmarkierung mit ^{125}I-desoxyridin. Strahlentherapie, 145, 161-170.

11. Begg, A.C., Sheldon, P.W. and Foster, J.L. (1974) Demonstration of radiosensitization of hypoxic cells in solid tumours by metronidazole. Brit. J. Radiol., 47, 399-404.

12. McNally, N.J. Denekamp, J., Sheldon, P.W. and Flockhart, I.R. (1978). Hypoxic cell sensitization by misonidazole in vivo and in vitro. Brit. J. Radiol., 51, 317-318.

13. Fowler, J.F., Sheldon, P.W., Denekamp, J. and Field, S.B. (1976) Optimum fractionation of the C3H mouse mammary carcinoma using X-rays, the hypoxic cell radiosensitizer Ro-07-0582, or fast neutrons. Int. J. Rad. Oncol. Biol. Phys., 1, 579-592.

14. Denekamp, J., Harris S.R., and Michael, B.D. (1974) Hypoxic cell radio-sensitizers: comparative tests of some electron affinic compounds using epidermal cell survival in vivo. Radiat. Res., 60, 119-132.

15. Foster, J.L. (pers. comm.)

16. Hendry, J.M. and Sutton, M.L. (1978) Care with radiosensitizers. Brit. J. Radiol. (in press).

17. Hirst, D.G. Vojnovic, B., Stratford, I.J. and Travis, E.L. (1978) The effect of the radiosensitizer misonidazole on motor nerve conduction velocity in the mouse. Brit. J. Cancer, 37, Supple. III, 237-241.

18. Denekamp, J., Fowler, J.F. and McNally, N.J. (1978) Hypoxic cell radiosensitizers: early or late in fractionated therapy? Brit. J. Cancer, 37, 858-860.

19. Denekamp, J. (1978) Cytotoxicity and radiosensitization in mouse and man. Brit. J. Radiol. 51, 636-637.

© 1979 Elsevier/North-Holland Biomedical Press
Radiosensitizers of Hypoxic Cells
A. Breccia, C. Rimondi and G.E. Adams eds.

KINETICS IN NEOPLASTIC PROLIFERATION AND INLFUENCE OF THERAPY.

G. PRODI

Istituto di Cancerologia, Università di Bologna, Bologna, Italy.

1. INTRODUCTION: THE VARIOUS LOGICAL BASES OF THERAPY.

The possibilities of intervention on the tumour are based upon several
"logical bases". They are different in that they act on distinct characteristics
of the neoplastic cells.

In the following, we shall be concerned only with medical types of
intervention (in the general meaning of "non-surgical").

There are three possible "logical bases", to which there correspond the
same number of methodologies.

a) The neoplastic cells is considered to be *a dividing cell*. The strategy of
intervention is based on interference with cell multiplication, and it
"selects" the neoplastic cells according to that characteristic. Since
neoplastic cells are not the only dividing cells in the organism, the
selectivity of this process is extremely limited. The therapeutic objective
is to increase it. This intervention strategy includes chemotherapy and
radiotherapy.

b) Neoplastic cells are *qualitatively different* from the normal cells of the
organism. Until now, only immunology (and not yet unequivocally) has permitted
the detection of qualitative differences and this has given rise to the approach
of immunotherapy.

Unfortunately, specific differences between neoplastic and normal cells
are limited, and there are not many ways of exploiting these differences in order
that the normal cells remain unaffected.

c) The neoplastic cell is considered to be a cell that is not very different
from the original cell. It has a residual differentiation, the characteristics
of which include mitotic regulability due to physiological factors. Therefore,
the logical basis of therapy in this case is the physiological interference with
proliferation.

152

Although in the future, results from the interference of the factors
of specific inhibition of the "calone" kind might be available, at present,
the regulation available is essentially hormonal, and is of use for tumours
of hormono-dependent organs which retain either completely or partially, their
hormono-dependence. The strategy resulting from this is hormonotherapy which
act on all the normal tissues affected by the endocrine action concerned.

The "selectivity" which makes possible the intervention is based upon the
magnitude of such parameter: for example the mitotic index, the immunogeniticity
with respect to the host and the level of residual hormono-dependence.

In this review we shall consider this first basis of therapy which is based
on the direct interference with cellular multiplication.

As an introduction we must examine tumour kinetics.

2. ELEMENTARY MODEL OF CELLULAR KINETICS IN TUMOURAL TISSUES.

Cells in tissues are generally subject to rigid mitotic regulation. For
simplicity, it can be said that cells are always potentially in proliferation,
and that therefore their regulation is inhibitory: total for stable elements,
partial for labile ones.

If a cellular element becomes insensitive to this regulation, and does not
respond to inhibitory stimuli, uncontrolled proliferation sets in. We shall
call this process "transformation and define "tumour" as the cellular expanding
population produced by it.

Let us consider an elementary model of neoplastic growth based on the
following hypotheses:

a) the tumour derives from a single cell;

b) the "switchin-off" of the inhibiting control is retained in all generations
after the first;

c) tumour growth is not in any way inhibited.

In this simple model, all cells divide continuously, and none of them
leave the tumour. The tumour is monoclonal and all tumour cells are identical
to the cell initially transformed.

If we accept these hypotheses, the tumour can be represented by simple

doubting kinetics in a plot it is represented by an exponential curve
(Fig. 1), or by a straight line if the scale of the ordinates (number of
cells) is logarithmic (Fig. 2).

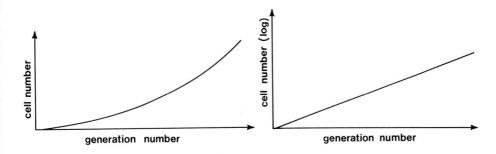

Fig. 1. Representation of tumour
cell number against generation
number (linear).

Fig. 2. Representation of tumour
cell number against generation
number (log.).

If the number of generations is plotted on the X-axis, a single curve
will show the trend of growth for all tumours. Since time it a more
convenient parameter than the number of generations and this is the parameter
that is actually measured, the various tumours show a different growth rate.
The various tumours can be represented by a group of straight lines
with different angular coefficients (Fig. 3).

The number of cells at time t is represented by the equation $N_t = N_o e^{kt}$.
K is a constant for a given tumour. The same consideration apply when
the growth of a tumour has to be expressed not in terms of the number
of its cells but by its weight. From the growth curve we obtain the doubling
period of the tumour. If we accept the hypothesis of this simple model,
the doubling period will coincide with the generation time, i.e.
with the lenght of the cellular cycle, as the population, and consequently

154

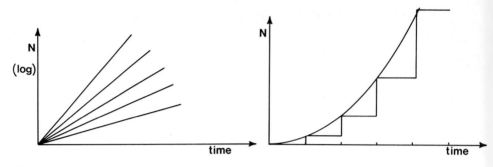

Fig. 3. Log N, cell number, against cell reproducing time for various tumours.

Fig. 4. Cell number (linear) growth in step-like tumoural growth

the weight and the volume, double at the same rate.

If the population were synchronized (which never actually occurs), tumour growth would be step-like, as is shown in the plot of Fig. 4. We can see that the number of the cells doubles in equal periods, and every "step" in the plot has twice the height of the previous one.

3. INFLUENCE OF THERAPEUTIC INTERVENTIONS ON THE SUGGESTED MODEL.

For a tumour corresponding to the hypotheses described above, a mitosis-inhibiting intervention can affect the growth curve in two ways:
a) the intervention is continuous (e.g. an antiproliferative drug kept at a constant concentration for the whole experiment). In this case, we can assume that on average the cycle length of each cell is increased (or the doubling period is increased, or the average number of generations per unit of time is decreased, and other equivalent expressions). The growth can always be represented by an exponential curve with a lower angular coefficient as for example, a change from curve (a) to curve (b) in Fig. 5.

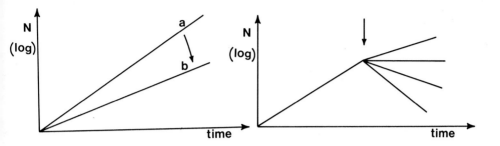

Fig. 5. Variation of cell growth during continuous intervention.

Fig. 6. Different inhibitory action on cell growth when intervention starts during the development of the tumour.

If the inhibitory action is strong, the straight line will coincide with the time-axis, the tumour will not grow. If the intervention starts at a certain stage of the development of the tumour, the slope will change in one of the ways shown in the plot, according to the effectiveness of the inhibitory action (Fig. 6).

The toxicity of the drug or radiation treatment obviously sets precise limits to the doses given.

b) The intervention is discontinuous (a single administration of one or more drugs or radiation). This is the normal case of therapy. The single intervention "eliminates" (i.e. sterilizes or kills, terms which we consider as equivalent at the moment) a number of cells in an exponential function of the dose.

E.g. if a dose removes 50% of the cells, two doses will remove 50% of the 50% left, and so on. It is easy to predict that, given the limitation of doses due to their toxicity, and the fact of operating on large numbers, it will not be possible to remove all the neoplastic cells with a single intervention. The remaining undamaged cells will start their growth again with their own kinetics. This can be shown in the plot of Fig. 7 where the arrow indicates the single intervention. The tumour is delayed by a period of time t_1-t_2 corresponding to the intervention.

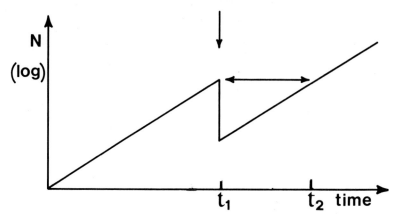

Fig. 7. Effects of successive interventions on tumour cell growth.

From this is derived the necessity of applying multiple discontinuous treatments (several administrations of drugs, several radiant interventions at fixed intervals) in order to reach a situations such as that represented in plot (a) (stationary condition) and in plot (b) (regression), as shown in Fig. 8a and 8b.

The considerations on the number of surviving cells, valid for the single intervention, also apply in the case of repeated intervention.

4. FURTHER CONDITIONS COMPLICATING THE ELEMENTARY MODEL: NON-PROLIFERATING FRACTION AND CELLULAR LOSS.

Few tumours only, and just for a short period, follow purely exponential kinetics as previously described. They are mainly experimental tumours, such as transplanted leukaemias, asciti tumours, etc.

It is necessary to take into account two factors which affecting the elementary model already described.

a) Not all the cells of the tumour multiply: some of them are at rest. There is therefore a non-proliferating fractions , which differs according to the tumour.

b) Not all dividing cells are retained within the tumour; a certain fraction of

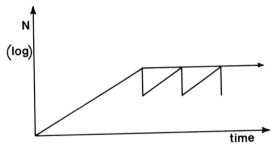

Fig. 8 a. Multiple discontinuous treatment which produces stationary conditions.

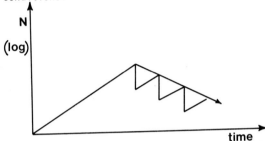

Fig. 8 b. Multiple discontinuous treatment which produces regression.

them is continuously lost, and leaves the system. Also this cellular loss differs from tumour to tumour.

In fact, the growth of a tumour is usually much slower than would be deduced from the duration of the mitotic cycle of the dividing cells. Some tumours made of components with high mitotic index can grow slowly, because only some of the neoplastic cells actually multiply, and other cells are continuously being lost (by necrosis, exfoliation, etc.). If these two quantities remain constant with time, and subtract from the growth a fraction constantly proportional to the neoplastic mass, the growth curve is always exponential, with an angular coefficient lower than that to be expected on the basis of the duration of the cycle of proliferating components. The effective period of real growth of the tumour is longer (sometimes much longer) than the cellular cycle of proliferating components. On the contrary if the cellular loss or a non-proliferating fraction undergoes sudden variations in time (e.g. for massive necrotic events), the growth curve will be irregular. The two quantities introduced (non-proliferating fraction and cellular loss) allow the

passage from the simplified exponential model described above to the
interpretation of real growth curves, obtainable from both experimental
and spontaneous tumours. In fact, the real doubling period of the tumour
can be measured by many techniques (direct or radiographic measurements,
counting the cellular elements, etc.).

This doubling period depends on the three components seen above:
overage duration of the cellular cycle of the proliferating fraction, extent
of cellular loss and the size of the non-proliferating fraction.

5. INFLUENCE OF THERAPY ON THE CELLULAR LOSS AND THE NON-PROLIFERATING FRACTION.

In section 3 the therapeutic intervention was schematized as an intervention
(continuous or discontinuous) exerting its influence on a homogeneous cellular
population totally in multiplication, thus prolonging the average period of
cellular generation. Through this the tumour is slowed down, without varying its
own general characteristics. In the more realistic description schematized in
the previous section, therapy can be considered, on the contrary, as an intervention accentuating one of the two factors interfering with the pure
exponential growth, i.e. the cellular loss and the non-proliferating fraction
(or both). So the growth of the tumour is seen as the overall outcome of the
input (of new cells), of the *output* (of old cells), and of the stationary
fraction, temporarily or definitively "sterile".

Even in the absence of therapeutic interventions, in many cases a balance
of the various quantities is attained so that, even in the case of highly
proliferating tumours, quite a slow growth results. With therapy, we can
obtain either a "killing" of cells that are eliminated sooner or later
(therefore there is an increase of cellular loss), or a "sterilization", i.e.
a passage of a certain amount of cells from the proliferating compartment
to the stationary sterile one. These two effects are not really distinct:
a first period of suspension of the growth of a certain cellular fraction,
achieved by the treatment, is followed by "recovery" (i.e. a return to the
proliferating compartment), or by death, i.e. by cellular loss.

In a homogeneous population, the probability that a single cell has of being damaged increases according to an exponential relation with the dose, as we have seen before. Also with different doses, in a large population, the probability of a certain number of cells avoiding the therapy is very high, and so the tumour could regain its growth curve starting from the surviving cells. According to the doses and the intervals between one dose and another, all possible combinations can be realised, from the slowing-down of growth to regression. Esperimentally, however, it is difficult to determine the contribution of both the non-proliferating fraction and cellular loss.

From a therapeutic point of view, the existence of a non-proliferating fraction is of great importance: the out-of-cycle cells are generally less vulnerable to treatment and have more time to repair the damage before an eventual resumption of the cycle. Therefore, the tumour with a non-proliferating fraction has a nearly treatment-proof cellular reserve that can return into the cycle.

Finally, also therapy can influence this state of affairs, in two opposite ways:
a) by eliminating part of the proliferating fraction, it can "recruit" (i.e. it can draw again into the cycle) part of the non-proliferating fraction. In this way, the effect of the therapy is partially cancelled, but, at the same time, some previously invulnerable cells become vulnerable to successive therapeutic interventions.
b) It can temporarily divert the proliferating fraction towards the non--proliferating fraction, inhibiting multiplication and increasing the out--of-cycle fraction. This makes the tumoural tissues less likely to be attacked by the next administration of drugs or radiations. These antagonistic effects vary from one tumour to another and from one drug to another, and many of their aspects are very little known.

These considerations underline the importance to be given to the schemes of therapy (distance between two administrations, association of several drugs, etc.), according to what will be clarified below.

6. VARIATIONS IN TIME OF THE DIFFERENT GROWTH PARAMETERS.

In the previous model we hypothesized that, in the presence of cellular loss and of a non-proliferating fraction constant in time, the kind of growth does not vary during the various phases of the tumour, and remains exponential. In effect, in most cases, the growth curve exhibits a slowing-down compared to the exponential growth of the first period. This slowing-down is regular in time too, and is well described by a Compertzian curve. It can be explained by the variation of all the parameters previously considered during the various phases of tumoural growth: the average duration of the cellular cycle becomes longer, the non-proliferating fraction increases, and the cellular loss can increase, too.

Let us examine schematically, the growth of a tumour transplantable in an animal, giving merely illustrative quantities (Fig. 9). The period from t_o to t_1 can be considered as exponential, according to what we have seen in the elementary model presented in section 2.

In this period, the proliferating fraction is 100%, there is no cellular loss, and the average generation time is (it is supposed) 24 hours. Between, t_1 and t_2 the generation time changes, e.g. to 30 hours, but this does not explain completely the slowing-down of growth: we can notice (the figures are again merely illustrative) that the proliferating fraction is not 100% but 80%. Between t_2 and t_3 the generation period becomes slightly longer (36 hours), but the proliferating fraction is lowered substantially to 60%.

The overall expansion of the tumour, due to a gradual variation of significant parameters, shows a slowing-down in comparison with a uniform growth of the exponential kind.

7. THERAPEUTIC CONSEQUENCES OF TIME VARIATIONS OF THE GROWTH PARAMETERS.

Time variations of the growth parameters suggests that there is a close relation between the natural history of the tumour and its treatment: the same treatment can have different effects in different phases of a tumour. More generally, since the therapeutic rationale we described in point 1 considers the cell to be neoplastic because it proliferates, the higher the mitotic index

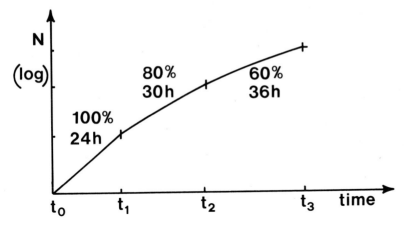

Fig. 9. Typical growth of a transplantable tumour.

of the tumour, the more effective will be the treatment. Consequently, the
same concentration of drug or the same dose of radiation is more effective
in the first development phases of the tumour, when all or almost all the
cells are in cycle, and the generation time is short. Later, the appearance
of a non-proliferating fraction and the slowing-down of the cycle lessen
its effectiveness.

This involves practical consequences of great interest:

a) Early diagnosis is important not only because it makes the estirpation
of the tumour possible before it infiltrates, but also because, from
a medical point of view, it allows a therapeutic intervention during the
most sensitive period.

b) The above considerations concerning the primary tumour are also valid
for metastasis. There is probably a starting phase of pure exponential growth
for each of them, when all the cells are in cycle; this cycle is clinically
silent.

The result is that the adjuvant post-surgical therapy (usually called
"metastasis-preventing") is justified also by kinetic considerations, as
it strikes the metastasis in the silent and more sensitive phase of micro-
metastasis: later it would be less effective.

8. HETEROGENEITY OF THE NEOPLASTIC POPULATION.

During the previous survey on the various models of increasing complexity, it was taken for granted that the tumoural population was homogeneous in time and space, and that the differences among the cells (e.g. in- and out-of-cycle cells) were merely functional and reversible. If we want a more realistic description of the tumour, we must introduce a further factor: heterogeneity. In most cases of malignant tumours, the overall population comprises subpopulations genetically different from one another.

Therefore, the growth characteristics of the tumour are the sum of the kinetics of a certain number of clones different from one another. Genetic heterogeneity depends upon a very significant parameter, the karyotype.

In malignant tumours, the karyotype is often aneuploid and widely dispersed. For example, there can be a majority line of 2N + x chromosomes (i.e. completely abnormal) close to many other minority lines of varying number, only occasional ly diploid. So the tumour is genetically heterogeneous, even if one particular population is the most responsible for its growth (a sort of stem line). The karyologic state (the plurality of subpopulations) is not stable with time. New clones appear, old clones disappear, minority clones prevail, the outline can change radically and the metastasis can show a different outline from that of the primitive tumour. These changes in time explain the so-called "progression", i.e. the evolution of the tumour towards an ever stronger malignancy; during its development, more autonomous, less immunogenetic clones, with a high mitotic index and less adjustable to physiologic conditions (less hormono-dependent), are selected.

Also in human pathology we can notice that, together with some tumours presenting the same growth characteristics during the whole of their natural history, there are others that undergo sudden changes, becoming unexpectedly invasive, increasing their mitotic index, etc. There are many examples of progression also in clinical practice.

9. THERAPEUTIC CONSEQUENCES OF THE HETEROGENEITY OF THE TUMOUR.

The relations between the heterogeneity of the neoplastic population

and medical therapy are very important, even if they are not usually
sufficiently underlined.

A drug acts on a homogeneous population in a homogeneous way. The
effect on a single cell is merely probabilistic and related to the dose,
every cell being, in this respect, equal to the others, i.e. not in
a preferential state. In the schemes presented above, a therapeutic condition
of all or nothing was hypothesized: a single cell is struck or not.
Only the chance of being struck varies with the dose. This scheme is
substantially exact. The situation of a heterogeneous population, however,
is different: the therapeutic intervention will affect the various populations
in various ways. Therefore, the consequences of a therapeutic intervention
are as follows.

a) The most sensitive populations are eliminated and the least sensitive
are favoured there by altering the global composition of the tumour.

b) Populations resisting the treatment are selected.

Heterogeneity is thus a favourable condition for the tumour because it
gives it the possibility of exploring new ways of survival in the surrounding
negative conditions imposed by the therapy.

We will not consider here the mechanism of the resistance to drugs and
radiation. However, it must be noticed that, because of the phenomena
of resistance, combined treatments both of polichemotherapy and of chemo and
radiotherapy are necessary in order to reduce to a minimum the probabilities
of selection of clones resistant to *all* the therapies used.

Resistance to *the same drug* can occur at different cellular levels
(e.g. modification of the entry at the level of the membrane, cytoplasmatic
metabolism of activation or inactivation etc.). Thus the ways in which
a cellular "mutant" acquires its resistance to a drug are many, and the
selection is a highly probabile event if we take into account that populations
of hundreds or thousands of millions of components are involved.

As a general consideration, we must stress the fact that we are obliged
to simplify the concept of tumour, presenting it as a total homogeneous
entity, whereas it is really the result of discrete and heterogeneous situations.

10. THE TUMOUR AS A STRUCTURE.

Up to now, we have considered the tumour as a cellular mass without any regular structure. We must make a further step in the "march towards reality" and consider its organization.

a) No matter how highly differentiated from the original tissue, a tumour always retains a memory of the organization of such tissue, and this can be seen not only at a morphologic level but also at the functional level. The fact is well-known, and allows the morphologic characterization (histologic and cytologic diagnosis, grading) and the functional characterization (determina tion of the hormono-dependence, of the differentiated production, etc.).

b) Only in the initial period can a tumour or a metastasis be considered as a mass of cells trophically maintained by diffusion. But soon the tumour becomes organized and a vascular component ensuring the blood supply can be seen in it. This means that the tumour acquires the blood vessels it needs by making and inductive action on the surrounding tissues. In effect the vasculo-stromal cells do not belong genetically to the tumour but to its host.

Therefore, the neoplastic tissue can exploit to its own advantage, residual inductive capacities, together with the sensitivity of host cells to such capacities. With regard to this, the tumour is not only aparasite imposing on its host, but also an interfering system directing the host's work to its own advantage. A tumoural tissue without the capacity to supply itself with blood vessels would be unable to exceed a given dimension; i.e. the dimension which permits feeding to occur through simple diffusion. Yet its morphogenetic capacity is not perfect: many observations of necrosis can be explained by an inadequate vascular network.

Within certain limits, then, it is improper to consider the tumour as an anarchic population. It is a structured tissue, even if only approximately and outside the organizing system of its host.

11. THERAPEUTIC CONSEQUENCES OF THE TUMOUR AS A STRUCTURE.

The morphogenetic-structural aspect can be considered from a therapeutic

point of view, analysing the influence of anti-mitotic therapy on vascularize
tion . This is a very important subject, even if scarcely investigated.

Briefly, these are the principal points:

a) The therapeutic intervention damages not only the neoplastic cells, but
also the blood vessels. A selective action in this direction could have
amplified consequences in comparison with the action directly carried out
on neoplastic cells. This happens in some interventions of radiotherapy
and chemoterapy, where necrotic and thrombotic effects due to vascular
damage appear, with a consequent fast alteration of the blood supply.

b) The vascularization of the tumour can be more or less efficient, and the
volume per minute can change from case to case.It is sometimes believed
that, in a tumour, a drug attains approximately the same concentration it
attains in serum, with the same kinetics. This is actually seldom the case.

If we inject a dye intravenously into an animal bearing a transplantable
tumour, and sacrifice it after a short time, we see that the tumour is lightly
and irregularly coloured. Therefore, a drug can sometimes not reach a sufficient concentration inside a tumour, or at least may reach it later and
for a shorter time.

If the drug has a short half-life, it can react with the normal tissues
completely before reacting with the tumoural tissue. The condition of
vascularization of a tumour, therefore, can cause a negative selectivity;
the normal tissues are, in that case, more damaged than the neoplastic tissue.
Generally, the conditions of vascularization of a tumour are extremely
important.

12. DAMAGE AND REPAIR.

In this paper which is focused on the kinetic aspects of the problem,
there is no emphasis on the mechanism of the mitotic cycle by itself, nor on
the mechanism of interference of radiation and drugs. Yet if we want to
understand the influence of therapeutic interventions on kinetics (in relation to the dose, and consequently, to the cellular loss and to the increase
of the non-proliferating fraction), we must consider the capacity of the cell

to repair the induced damage. Therefore, it is advisable to say a few words
on some basic points.

a) Radiation and antimitotics do not have a preferential target. They induce
damage where there are suitable chemicophysical conditions (interaction of
the radiation or of the drugs with the macromolecules). So proteins, poly-
saccharides, RNA, DNA etc. are affected in ways which differ from case to
case. Yet it is the sort of structure affected that "selects" the significant
damage; with normal doses, the damage induced on the macromolecules present
in many copies in the cells is not very important, as they are continuously
renewed and replaceable. On the contrary, the damage induced on a "single
copy" structure is very important, as it can only be replaced by a duplication
which perpetuates the damage, i.e. DNA. That is why we usually say that
DNA is the specific target of radiation and antimitotics.

b) The various drugs and radiation are effective during the whole cycle,
during only one phase of the cycle and also on the out-of-cycle cells. There
is a large range of possibilities, according to the type of therapeutic
intervention. However, it is during the multiplication that the damage is
made evident. Hence, even for non-cyclo-specific interventions (which can
affect the DNA during all phases, even in Go), it is necessary for the cells
to multiply.

c) The cells are provided with enzymatic systems capable of detaching the
DNA sections altered by the treatment, replacing them with segments copied
according to the normal information present in the other filament.

   Therefore the damage is not only related to the drug concentration or
to the dose of radiations (hence to the intensity of the damage), but also
to the repairing capacity of a cell - i.e. to the effectiveness of the enzymatic
systems in question.

d) Since the repairing system has its own kinetics, a cell affected during
phase S will have little time to repair the damage, whereas a cell quiescent
in Go will have more time (hence the attempt to affect the population selectively through cell synchronization and chronologically defined administration of the treatment). Thus a cell affected during or just before

phase S has more probability of transferring the damage to the daughter cells, in this way making it impossible for the damage to be repaired, as it has become a sequence error, i.e. an informational alteration.

e) Data on the real repairing capacity of DNA in various kinds of tumours are still rather scarce. At least hypothetically, it can be said that selectivity (through which, in relation to the normal proliferating cells, the tumour is sometimes really affected more than would be expected), is due to the weaker repairing capacity of the neoplastic tissue, and therefore to its weaker general recovery. This is shown in the diagram in Fig. 10 where the dashed line represents a normal proliferating tissue and the continuous line the neoplastic tissue.

If a certain treatment at time t_o depresses both by the same amount (as we can see at time t_1), at time t_2 the normal tissue is already restored, but the tumoural tissue is not. Repeating the treatment when the tumour tissue is still depressed at time t_2, t_3 etc., only the tumoural tissue is progressively depressed.

13. THERAPEUTIC CONSEQUENCES OF DAMAGE AND REPAIR.

Damaging the DNA is of course what therapy tries to accomplish. Without dwelling too much on this point, since we are mostly interested in kinetics, we will nevertheless examine three problems in this context.

a) The damage, in some cases, can be directed selectively at its target. As far as radiation is concerned, the techniques for directing most of the dose at a tumour rather than at the neighbouring normal tissues, are numerous and well-known. As far as drugs are concerned, techniques of local perfusion are used in some cases. Attempts are also being made to convey drugs to the tumour by means of antitumoural antibodies, or by means of phagocytotic particles in the case of tumours with a phagocytotic properties. However, results are still scarce.

b) The damage can be increased or reduced by concomitant interventions. As far as radiotherapy is concerned, radioprotectors reduce the effect, and the whole range of radio-sensitizing substances (which are the subject

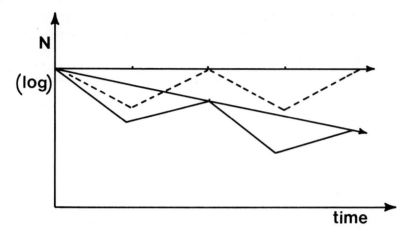

Fig. 10. Cel growth of a normal proliferating tissue (dashed line) and of a neoplastic tissue (continuous line).

of this course) and even oxygen increase the effect.

It is important to establish whether some of these drugs can be selectively concentrated in neoplastic cells, thus increasing the damage. It may be possible that the cellular membrane in some tumours is more permeable towards some of them, that they are kept longer, or metabolized more slowly. It is likewise important to assess whether the increase of the damage caused can be interpreted as a greater effectiveness of the break down of DNA.

c) Up to now, the occurrence of inhibition of repairing systems is completely unknown, even though it is of great theoretical and practical importance. For example, if we apply local action through radiation and at the same time administer intravenously a substance able to inhibit repair the local damage is increased. Hitherto, the substances considered as repair inhibitors (caffeine, phorbalesters, some steroids) are shown to be aspecific, or anyhow, not sufficiently selective. It is possible that some radiosensitizing substances can act by inhibiting repair of the DNA. A great deal of basic and applied research is needed in this field.

14. CONCLUSIONS: THERAPEUTIC MODELS.

Animal systems are important reference points in antineoplastic experimenta
tion . Whoever is active in this research field must pay attention to
some strange discrepancies between animal systems and clinical situations. On
one hand, some experimental models are extremely optimistic: in some
experimental leukaemias, for example, chemotherapy achieves rapid recoveries
which are not realizable in human leukaemias. On the other hand, good results
are sometimes obtained in the clinic, (e.g. in Hodgkin's disease, corionepithe
lioma etc.), without any experimental support. There are two points of
view on this subject, or rather, two tactics to follow: we can defend a
strict experimental attitude by conducting the whole experimentation cycle on
the animal and only at the end passing to clinical cases, or we can
adopt original therapeutic schems on man, making some variation on the basis
of experience.

In effect, these are not two opposite points of view and they must be com
plementary to one another. We obviously cannot pass into clinical use without
some basic experimental facts acquired from animals, but also we cannot expect
animal tumours to reflect the complex situations presented by human tumours.

Also if differences on the treatment between animals and man can be
achieved studing the kinetic of neoplastic proliferation, in the application
of radiosensitizing drug of hypoxic cell kinetic studies are . . of scarce
interest at the present knowledge of their mechanism of action.

In fact the growth of V 79 - 379 A cell is affected only at higher concentration than used for therapeutic treatment (I.J. Stratford and G.E. Adams,
1977)[1]. In a previous work Asquite et al. (1974)[2] found that the sensitizing
ability of misonidazole is entireles indipendent of the position of
the cell in the mitotic cycle; the same surviving fraction was obtained
by a single enhancement ratio et all points in the cell cycle.

This parallels previous demonstration that both oxygen and some other
electron affinic compounds sensitize hypoxic V 79 cells equally at all stages
of the cycle.

These kinds of research in vitro have not been yet confirmed in vivo,

animals and man, mostly with respect with the immunological reaction
of the tissue.

For this if in the future we want to realize an average effective therapy,
that makes possible the use of all the resources at our disposal,
our preliminary objective must be the individual definition of the tumour,

not only of its morphological characteristics, but also, of its functional
parameters in connection with a few basic points: 1) kinetic characteristics
concerning proliferation, but not for radiation and hypoxic cell sensitizers
treatment, 2) determination of the hormonodependence, 3) determination of
the immunogeneticity in relation to the host. Whilst this last point
is not yet resolved the first two have already given interesting results.

REFERENCES

1. I.J. Stratford and G.E. Adams, Br. J. Cancer, 35, 307, 1977.
2. J.C. Asquite, M.E. Watts, K. Patel, C.E. Smithen and G.E. Adams, Radiat. Res., 60, 108, 1974.

GENERAL BIBLIOGRAPHY

Baserga R., Editor, The Cell Cycle and Cancer, DEKKER, New York, 1971.

Baserga R., Editor, Multiplication and Division in Mammalian Cell, DEKKER, New York, 1976.

Bresciani F., Cell Proliferation in Cancer, Eur. J. Cancer, 4, 389, 1968.

Dethlefsen L.A., Prewitt J.M.S., Mendhelsohn M.L.: Analysis of Tumour Growth Curve, J. Natl. Cancer Inst., 40, 389, 1968.

Fried J., Proposal for the Determination of Generation Time Variability and Dormancy of Proliferating Cell Populations, J. Theor. Biol. 34, 535, 1970.

Laird A.K., Dynamics of Tumour Growth, Br. J. Cancer 19, 278, 1965.

Lala P.K., in "Methods in Cancer Research" vol. 6, H. Busch, Editor, Academic Press, New York.

Lammerton F. and Fray R.J.M. editors, Cell Proliferation, Blackwell, Oxford, 1963.

Lightdale C. and Lipkin M., "Cell Division and Tumour Growth", Cancer vol. 3, Becker F.F. editor, Plenum Press, New York, 1975.

Mendelsohn M.L., "The Kinetics of Tumour Cell Proliferation" in Cellular Radiation Biology, Williams and Wilkins, Baltimore, 1965.

Prodi G., La Biologia dei Tumori, chap. 1,2,3, CEA, Milano 1977.

Rajewsky M.F., Handbuch der Allgemeinen Pathologie, VI/5, Springer.

Simpson-Herren L. and Lloyd H.H. Kinetic Parameters and Growth Curves for Experimental Tumour Systems, Cancer Chemother. Rep., $\underline{54}$, 143, 1970.

Steel G.G., Cell Loss as a Factor in the Growth Rate of Human Tumours, Eur. J. Cancer $\underline{3}$, 381, 1967.

Steel G.G., The Cell Cycle in Tumours, Cell Tissue Kinet. $\underline{5}$, 87, 1972.

Tubiana M., The Kinetics of Tumour Cell Proliferation and Radiotherapy, Brit. J. Radiol. $\underline{44}$, 325, 1971.

© 1979 Elsevier/North-Holland Biomedical Press
Radiosensitizers of Hypoxic Cells
A. Breccia, C. Rimondi and G.E. Adams eds.

HEAVY PARTICLE METHODS OF SENSITIZING HYPOXIC CELLS

JACK F. FOWLER

Gray Laboratory of Cancer Research Compaign, Mount Vernon Hospital, Northwood, Middlesex, HA6 2RN, England.

INTRODUCTION

There are three radiobiological differences between low LET [*] and high LET radiation.

(1) There is less repair of sublethal radiation damage after high LET radiation.[1]

(2) The oxygen enhancement ratio (OER) is smaller for high LET radiation (Fig. 1).[2]

(3) There is less difference in radiosensitivity for the different phases of the cell cycle for high LET radiation.[3]

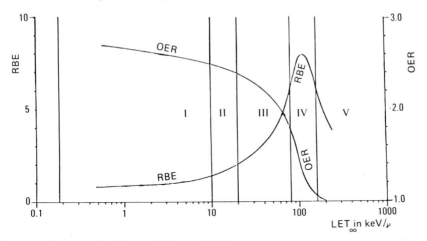

Fig. 1. Changes in OER and RBE as LET increases.

[*] Linear Energy Transfer (LET) denotes the density of ionization and excitation along the track of a charged particle. It is the rate of loss of energy of the particle, in keV per micron of track length. Low LET radiation (electrons, X-rays gamma-rays) have LET values between 0.2 and about 10 keV/um. If the G-value is 4.5 for the production of free electrons in water this corresponds to about 10-150 ion pairs per micron. High LET radiation includes protons (released in tissue by neutrons) and heavier charged particles accelerated in cyclotrons, synchrontrons or linear accelerators.

The first difference may or may not be useful in radiotherapy, depending
on whether it is greater for the tumour than the normal tissues. This will
vary from one type of tumour to another and more research is required on
this aspect.

The second difference provides the major gain expected for high LET beams.
It will obviously be an advantage for any tumours which contain a significant
proportion of hypoxic cells. They will be less protected by hypoxia, in relation
to well-oxygenated tissues, than when X-rays are used.

The third difference would be an advantage in the treatment of any tumours
having a high proportion of cells in S-phase (i.e. dividing) than the irradiated
normal tissues have, because cells in S-phase are most resistant to low LET
radiation. This is a likely occurrence but we do not know whether the very
slowly turning-over tissues in which late injury is important are normally
in a state which may also be resistant to low LET radiation. If so the advantage
would not exist.

Therefore the greater relative effect on hypoxic cells is the main advantage
expected for high LET radiotherapy.

PHISICAL DEPTH DOSE CHARACTERISTICS

Figure 2 shows the relative depth doses of cobalt-60, fast neutrons, 20 MeV
betatron photons, protons, protons and negative pi mesons. The fast neutrons

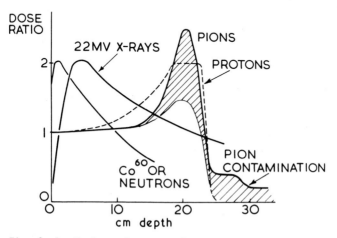

Fig. 2. Depth doses for several types of radiotherapy beam.

and pions are high LET particles but cobalt-60, betatron photons and accelerated protons are not. In the case of pions there is the double advantage of an ideal physical dose distribution together with high LET radiation in the "peak". At the end of each pion track, the negative pi meson is attracted into a nucleus and causes it to explode ("nuclear star") giving off alpha particles, neutrons, protons, and a few heavier nuclei.

Accelerated protons however have the same radiobiological properties as low LET radiation (except in the final fraction of a millimetre of their track). Their advantage is therefore purely that of the physical dose distribution.

Other heavy ions can also be accelerated and used for radiotherapy, notably at Berkeley, California, where accelerated neon ions are just starting to be used for radiotherapy. These particles have a high LET for the final few centimetres of their track (Table 1) so they, like pions, combine the advantages of a good physical depth dose with those of high LET in the target region.

TABLE 1

DISTANCE ALONG TRACK FOR WHICH LET_{oo} CAN EXCEED:

Ion	50 keV/um	100 keV/um
ARGON	100 cm	10 cm
NEON	6	1
NITROGEN	1.6	0.3
CARBON	0.8	0.15
HELIUM	0.02	0.01
PROTON	0.01	0.01

(Reduced by straggling and collision)

In the superficial layers of tissue, traversed by the "plateau" region of the incoming particles, the radiation is low LET, because the particles are travelling too fast to be at high LET. Therefore multiple small doses would permit the same recovery between fractions that is found in conventional low-LET radiotherapy. Less recovery however occurs in the "peak" region of pions and heavy particles so that the RBE is higher there, adding to the physical dose advantage in the peak relative to the plateau.

Both pions and heavy charged particles are unavoidably contaminated with low LET particles in their high-dose peaks. The pion "stars" provide fast protons, which are low LET, and the peak also includes about half its dose as the low-LET track of incoming pions (the part under the shading in Fig. 2). The heavy charged particle beams are unavoidably contaminated with their own delta rays, which are fast electrons branching off the main particle track. Therefore the RBE's are not as high and the OER's are not as low as had once been hoped. The values of OER are 1.6-1.8, similar to those of neutrons or even marginally higher, which is less advantageous for radiotheraphy.[4]

Neutrons therefore provide the fullest advantages of high LET radiation from the radiobiological point of view. However, their depth doses are poor. In Fig. 2 they are shown as having the same depth dose as cobalt-60 radiation. Even this can only be achieved by cyclotrons producing deuterons of energy at least 35 MeV, which are expensive. The smaller deuterium-tritium machines, which produce mono-energetic neutrons of 14 MeV energy, do not yield very high dose rates and have rather large penumbra. At present cyclotrons are the most popular sources of neutrons. Some ten or twelve are in clinical use or planned. About eight 14 MeV D-T generators are in use or planned, throughout the world.

DEPENDENCE OF RBE ON DOSE PER FRACTION

Figure 3 shows cell survival curves for a series of particle beams of increasing LET.[5] The larger shoulder on the lower LET curves means that the RBE's are larger for low doses (less degree of cell kill) than for higher doses.

Figure 4 shows measured values of neutron RBE for various normal tissues.[6] The increase of RBE with decrease in dose is obvious for each tissue. There are differences in the RBE values for these normal tissues.

EFFECTS OF NEUTRONS ON EXPERIMENTAL TUMOURS

Figure 5 shows the corresponding results for animal tumours of various

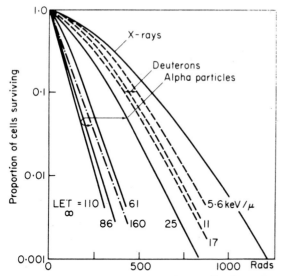

Fig. 3. Cell survival curves for radiation of several LET values.

types.[7] Where these RBE's are higher than those for normal tissues, there is obviously a therapeutic advantage in using neutrons. At the low doses appropriate to multifraction radiotherapy however, about 100 rads per fraction, data are few.

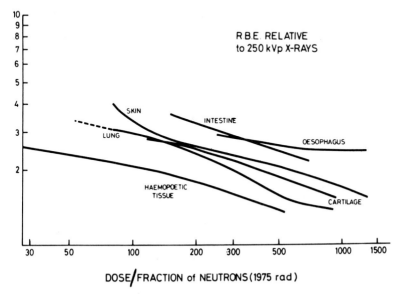

Fig. 4. RBE versus neutron dose per fraction (log-log plot).

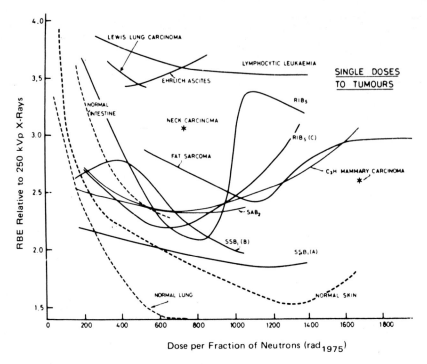

Fig. 5. RBE versus neutron dose per fraction for humans.

Figure 6 shows the results of fractionated radiotherapy studies on the C3H mouse mammary carcinoma[8] already described in Figures 4 and 5 of my other paper in the present Course. The vertical bars represent the results for cyclotron neutrons. Other symbols are for X-rays only. The proportion of tumours locally controlled is plotted at the dose which causes the same acute skin reaction for each schedule. Although the spread of results for neutrons is greater than it was for hypoxic-cell radiosensitizers and X-rays, the tendency is the same. The single-dose results are greatly improved. Two fractions are also improved. At the optimum overall time the improvement may or may not be significant.

The single-dose results were improved to the same extent as when misonidazole was added to X-rays. This would be expected because both the SER and the neutron gain factor* were 1.7.

---

* OER for X-rays divided by OER for neutrons. This ratio usually comes out at about 1.7 (1.6-1.8) for cells of several types and neutrons of various energies in the range used for therapy.

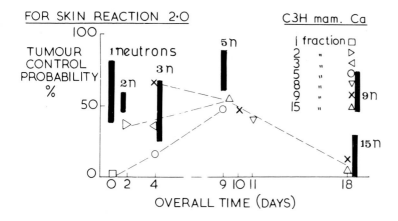

Fig. 6. Tumours cure, at constant skin reaction, for various fractionation schedules. ,0, X - Xrays only. Bars-Neutrons.

Figure 7 shows results for another type of tumour.[9] Again the results are plotted as effect on tumours (delay in regrowth) for a constant degree of acute skin reaction. The points X show that for X-rays only an increased tumour delay was obtained by dividing the treatment into 2 or 5 fractions with 48-hour intervals between each. The points 0 show the improvements when misonidazole was given before each X-ray dose. The points N show the results when cyclotron neutrons alone were used. The gain is the same for

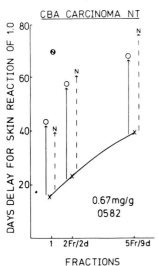

neutrons as for misonidazole at the concentrations used. When misonidazole was used together with neutrons, the result shown at 0 was obtained for single doses. It was better than for neutrons alone or for X-rays with misonidazole, as would be expected because both these modalities yielded gain factors of only 1.7 instead of the full OER of 2.5-3. When misonidazole was used with 2 or 5 fractions of neutrons, smaller gains were observed[9]; not shown here.

Fig. 7. X - Xrays only; N - Neutrons only; 0 - Xrays + Ro-0582.

The use of 6 or 25 fractions of X-rays each with misonidazole should give
SER values of 1.6-1.7 or 1.3-1.4 respectively. These are to be compared with
the neutron gain factors of 1.6-1.8. It is clear that misonidazole is able
at high doses, but not quite at low doses, to equal the advantage provided
by fast neutrons.

When multiple doses of neutrons are used, the measured gain factors also
fall to values of 1.1-1.3, depending on type of tumour. This is partly due
to reoxygenation in the tumours, so that the measured gain is the most that
could be achieved by any method, even if it were more powerful at eliminating
hypoxic cells than the agents used.

In summary, neutrons can at present provide a slightly greater advantage
than misonidazole at the concentrations which it is possible to use clinically.
However, the upper limits of the expected effect of misonidazole on hypoxic
cells overlap the lower limits of those expected from neutrons. When used
together, misonidazole and neutrons give a bigger advantage than neutrons alone
or misonidazole with X-rays, for single doses or up to 5 fractions. Further
information is required on the results of all these modalities for multiple
small fractions.

CLINICAL RESULTS OF NEUTRON THERAPY

Animal experiments using pigs[10,10a] showed that the severe late normal-tissue
complications reported by Stone[11] could be avoided, provided that the increase
in neutron RBE with decrease in dose per fraction was allowed for (Sheline
et al.[12]).

Dr. Catterall and her colleagues at Hammersmith Hospital have used the
MRC cyclotron (16 MeV deuterons on beryllium) to carry out a trial of neutron
therapy on very advanced cancer of the head and neck. Figure 8 summarises the
results[13,14]. The local control of tumours was increased from 19% to 76%
using neutrons instead of photons, a large and highly significant increase.
This increase remains equally big, and still significant, if all the patients
treated with somewhat low doses of photons are excluded from the analysis.
Table II shows this and provides a clear answer to some critics of this
clinical trial.

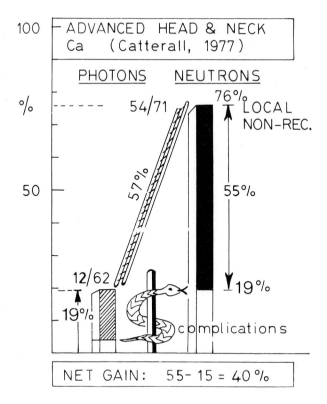

Fig. 8. Results of clinical trials at Hammersmith.

However there was also an increase in severe complications from 4% to 19%; this is the real criticism of the trial. Some of the neutron complications may be attributed to the fixed horizontal beam with less good physical penetration than cobalt-60 and others to the fact that these very advanced tumours had eaten away large volumes of normal tissue. It remains to be shown whether a neutron beam of *good* physical properties, comparable in depth dose to conventional megavoltage photon therapy machines, can maintain such a dramatic increase in local control as shown in Fig. 8 with less increase in normal tissue complications.

Although these clinical results represent one of the largest improvements in local tumour control obtained in any clinical trial, they do not yet prove that neutrons are better than photons. This proof will require a trial where

TABLE II

FAST NEUTRON CLINICAL TRIAL ADVANCES HEAD AND NECK Ca.

		PROTONS	NEUTRONS	P
(1)	Local Control (All patients)	12/62 (19%)	54/71 (76%)	.001
(2)	Hammersmith patients only	5/25 (20%)	18/20 (90%)	.001
(3)	Patients receiving 110-130 TDF only	3/12 (25%)	53/68 (78%)	.01
(4)	Patients receiving 110-120 TDF only	3/11 (27%)	30/37 (81%)	.024
(5)	Serious complicns. in normal tissues	2/45 (4%)	12/58 (17%)	.02
(6)	Complicns. as a propn. of patients with controlled primaries	2/11 (18%)	12/47 (26%)	Not Sig.

the normal tissue complications are not significantly different in the neutron
and photon groups. Further trials are in progress in some 20 centres in at
least eight countries. More penetrating neutron beams are required for the
next stage of clinical trials. A cyclotron and moving-beam isocentric head
for this would cost about £1M and the complete installation just less than
£2M. Costs of other particle accelerators will be discussed further below.

NEGATIVE PI MESONS AND HEAVY PARTICLES

Pions have the double advantage of a peak in depth dose and high LET in
the peak. They are already being used clinically at Los Alamos, U.S.A.[15] and
will be used at Villigen, near Zurich, Switzerland and at Vancouver, Canada.
Heavy particles have the same double advantage. Accelerated neon particles
are just beginning to be used clinically at Berkeley, California. If these
types of beam give good clinical results, we shall not know whether it is

because of the good physical dose distribution or because of the biological advantages of high LET. They are the most expensive of the beams of radiation proposed for radiotherapy.

PROTON BEAMS

Protons (of 180-200 MeV) have the physical advantage of the peak at a depth in tissue but they are radiobiologically the same as low LET radiation. They are being used to treat deep-seated cancer at Boston, U.S.A. and Moscow, U.S.S.R. There is also some experience of this at Uppsala, Sweden[16].

If the results of the proton beams are good, this would indicate that the physical advantage of the more expensive heavier particles or pions is the important advantage. If however results of the neutron beams are good, this would indicate that the physical advantage of the peak is unimportant and that the better radiobiological effect of the high LET is the main advantage. We cannot interpret the pion results without those from protons on one hand and neutrons on the other.

It is logical to suggest applying hypoxic-cell sensitizers to proton beams. This would provide ideal physical depth doses more cheaply than from pions or heavy particles, together with the main radiobiological advantage expected from high LET, the ability to eliminate hypoxic cells.

RELATIVE COSTS

It was stated above that the cost of a 40-45 MeV cyclotron to produce a neutron beam better than cobalt-60 in penetration would be about £1M ($2M). The sequence of increasing costs of accelerators is: neutrons, protons, heavy particles, pions[17]. Each step requires just less than a doubling in cost of the machine required. Costs of buildings would be extra. There are no problems of dose rate for protons or heavy particles because the primary particle beams are used. Pions however are secondary particles, usually from a beam of 500-800 MeV protons, so that very high proton currents are required to provide useful dose rates. Few pion generators are likely in any one country.

CONCLUSIONS

The main radiobiological advantage from high LET beams is expected to be the relatively greater effect on hypoxic cells. This may not be the only advantage but the others are less well substantiated. Misonidazole, with its known limitation of clinical dose level, gives nearly as large an effect on hypoxic cells as high LET radiation, but not quite as large. Misonidazole together with neutrons gave a larger gain in experimental tumours than either neutrons alone or X-rays plus misonidazole, although further research on the effects of multiple small fractions is necessary. If hypoxic-cell sensitizers were used with proton beams the advantages both of an ideal physical depth dose and the extra effect on hypoxic cells would be obtained, more cheaply than with heavier ions or pions.

ACKNOWLEDGEMENTS

I have pleasure in thanking past and present colleagues for stimulating discussions and allowing me to quote their data as referenced. I also thank the editors of Radiation Research Quarterly for Figs. 1, 4 and 5; Cancer in Ontario 1976 for Fig. 2; Academic Press, Inc., for Fig. 3; British Journal of Radiology for Figs. 6 and 8; Atomkern energie for Fig. 7.

REFERENCES

1. Fowler, J.F. and Morgan, R.L. (1963) Pre-therapeutic experiments with the fast neutron beam from the Medical Research Council Cyclotron. VIII General Review. Brit. J. Radiol., 36, 115-121.

2. Barendsen, G.W., Koot, C.J., van Kersen, G.R., Bewley, D.K., Field, S.B. and Parnell, C.J. (1966) The effect of oxygen on impairment of the proliferative capacity of human cells in culture by ionizing radiations of different LET. Int. J. Rad. Biol., 10, 317-327.

3. Hall, E.J. (1969) Radiobiological measurements with 14 MeV neutrons. Brit. J. Radiol., 42, 805-813.

4. Rayu, M.R. and Richman, C. (1972) Negative Pion radiotherapy: physical and radiobiological aspects. Curr. Topics Radiat. Res. Quart., 8, 159-233.

5. Barendsen, G.W., Walter, H.M.D., Fowler, J.F. and Bewley, D.K. (1963) Effects of different ionizing radiations on human cells in tissue culture. Radiat. Res., 18, 106-119.

6. Field, S.B. and Hornsey, S. (1971) RBE values for cyclotron neutrons for effects on normal tissues and tumours as a function of dose and dose fractionation. Europ. J. Cancer, 7, 161-169.

7. Field, S.B. (1976) An historical survey of radiobiology and radiotherapy with fast neutrons. Curr. Topics Radiat. Res. Quart., 11, 1-86.

8. Fowler, J.F., Sheldon, P.W., Denekamp, J. and Field, S.B. (1976) Optimum fractionation of the C3H mouse mammary carcinoma using X-rays, the hypoxic-cell radiosensitizer Ro-07-0582, or fast neutrons. Int. J. Rad. Oncol., Biol., Phys., 1, 579-592.

9. Denekamp, J., Morris, C. and Field, S.B. (1977). The response of a trans-planted tumour to fractionated irradiation. III - Fast neutrons plus the radiosensitizer Ro-07-0582. Radiat. Res., 70, 425-432.

10. Bewley, D.K., Fowler, J.F., Morgan, R.L., Silvester, J.A. and Turner,B.A. (L963) VII. Experiments on the skin of pigs with fast neutrons and 8 MV X-rays, including some effects of dose fractionation. Brit. J. Radiol., 36, 107-115.

11. Stone, R.S. (1948) Neutron therapy and specific ionization. Am. J. Roentgenol., 59, 771.

12. Sheline, G.E., Phillips, T.L., Field, S.B., Brennan, J.T. and Raventos, A. (1971) Effects of fast neutrons on human skin. Am. J. Boentgenol., 111, 31-41.

13. Catterall, M., Sutherland, I. and Bewley, D.K. (1975) First results of a randomized clinical trial of fast neutrons compared with X or gamma rays in treatment of advanced tumours of the head and neck. Brit. Med. Jour., 21 June, 653-656.

14. Catterall, M., Bewley, D.K. and Sutherland, I. (1977). Second report on results of a randomised clinical trial of fast neutrons compared with X or gamma rays in treatment of advanced tumours of head and neck. Brit. Med. Jour., 25 June, 1642-1643.

15. Kligerman, M.M., Sala, J.M., Wilson, S. and Yuhas, J.M. (1978) Investiga-tion of pion-treated human skin nodules for therapeutic gain. Int. J. Radiat. Oncol., Biol., Phys., 4, 263-265.

16. Suit, H.D., Goitein, M., Tepper, J.E., Verhey, L., Koehler, A.M., Schneider, R. and Gragoudas, E. (L977) Clinical experience and expectations with helium and heavy ion irradiation. Int. J. Radiat.Oncol., Biol., Phys., 3, 115-126.

17. Grunder, A. and Leeman, C.W. (1977) In "Report on Biological & Medical Research with Accelerated Heavy Ions at the Bevalac 1974-77". Lawrence Berkeley Laboratory Report No. LBL-5610, p. 223.

Radiosensitizers of Hypoxic Cells
A. Breccia, C. Rimondi and G.E. Adams eds.

187

ANALYTICAL TECHNIQUES APPLIED TO THE STUDY OF RADIOSENSITIZING DRUGS AND OF THEIR METABOLITES

E. GATTAVECCHIA

Istituto Chimico, Facoltà di Farmacia, Università degli Studi di Bologna, Bologna (Italy)

INTRODUCTION

The sensitizing effect of a given drug is directly related to its concentration in the irradiated site[1], and consequently it is important to know the kinetics both with respect to its metabolic stability and its rate of penetration in order to optimize treatments and obtain maximum effectiveness. It is desirable that the radiosensitizer should diffuse unchanged into the tissue prior to the irradiation even if, in some cases, the products of drug metabolism are still active in cellular sensitization[2].

It is relevant in this respect to know the kinetics of absorption, distribution and elimination of the drugs from a patient according to the following scheme:

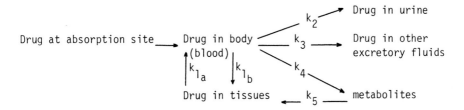

Present interest is focused mainly on nitroimidazole derivatives as radiosensitizers of hypoxic cells[3]. In particular 1-ethanol-2-methyl-5-nitroimidazole, (I°, metronidazole or flagyl) and 1-(3-methoxy), propan-2, ol -2-nitroimidazole (II°, misonidazole or Ro 07-0582) have been investigated to some extent. Knowledge of the transformation mechanisms of the major metabolites of these compounds, and of techniques applicable for their identification and analysis is very useful in investigations on the utilization of these drugs.

METABOLISM OF NITROIMIDAZOLES

Although the metabolism of a certain drug may vary from person to person, the main metabolic route for nitroimidazole derivatives consists of oxidation of the side chain. Stambaugh and coworkers[4] have shown that the metabolic process for metronidazole follows the scheme in Fig. 1.

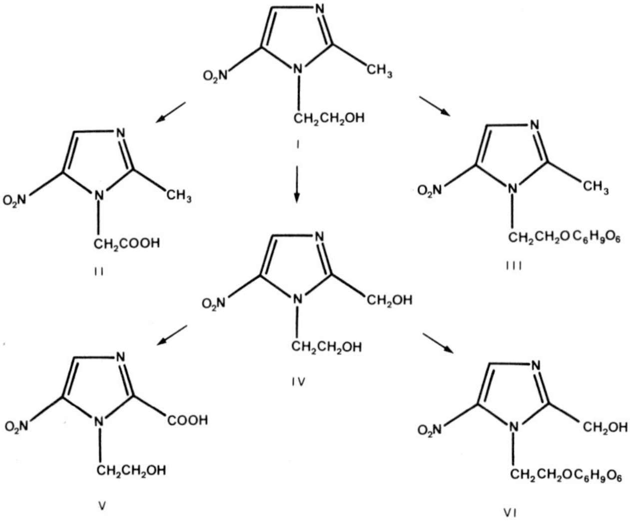

Fig. 1. Metabolic behaviour of metronidazole.

The compounds that are frequently expelled in the urine are metronidazole and its ether conjugated with glucoronic acid. (I+III 30-40%) and 1-(2--hydroxyethyl)2-hydroxymethyl -5-nitroimidazole together with its conjugated ether (IV+VI 40-50%). The reduction of the nitro group does not seem to occur to any appreciable extent, although the presence in the urine of an azocompound probably deriving from condensation of partially reduced Flagyl molecules, has been detected[5].

The metabolism of misonidazole leads mainly to formation of its o-de-methylated derivative (which has been shown to be a radiosensitizer in vitro[6]) and, in small quantities, to the normation of an amino derivative[7], Fig. 2.

Also another 2-nitroimidazole, such as DL347, Lepetit (1 methyl-5-(1-methyl

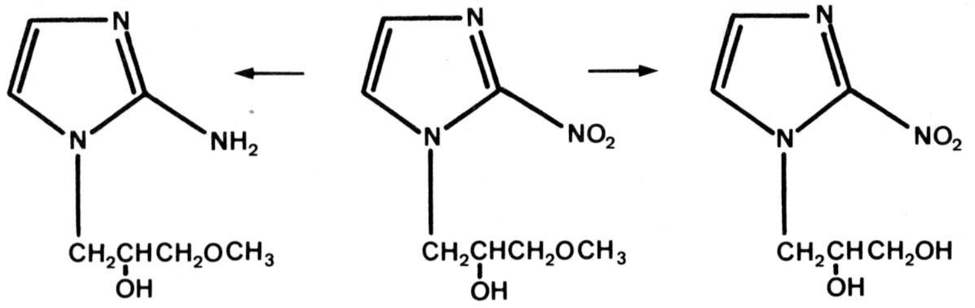

Fig. 2. Metabolic behaviour of misonidazole.

ethyl)-2-nitroimidazole) show oxidative metabolism[8,9] at the side chain, see Fig. 3.

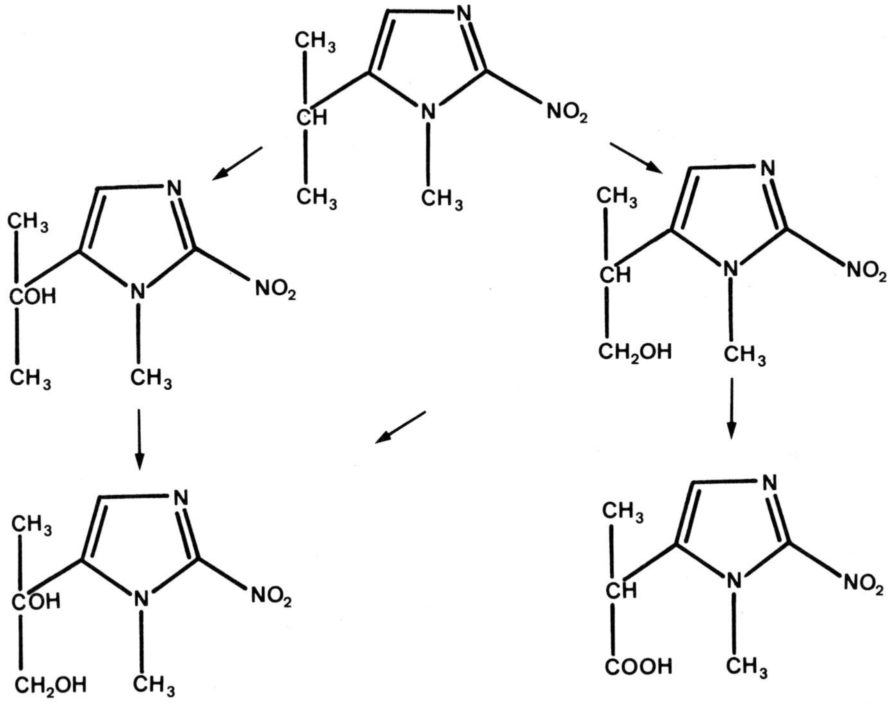

Fig. 3. Metabolic oxidation of 1-methyl-5-(1-methylethyl) 2-nitroimidazole.

Dosage techniques

The analytical techniques which are best suited for the determination of nitroimidazole derivates in biological tissues and fluids are mainly polarography, UV and visible spectrophotometry, paper chromatography (PC), thin layer chromatography (TLC), gas chromatography (GC) and high pressure liquid chromatography (HPLC).

In general, an analytical technique often calls for three steps:

a) separation

b) identification

c) quantitative determination,

although these three steps are not always necessary and do not always consist of three distinct operations.

Polarography

This technique is sufficiently simple and sensitive (the lowest quantity detectable of metronidazole is 0.1 μg/mL) and can be directly applied to the analysis of serum and plasma. The height of the polarographic wave (or the peak in the case of pulse-polarography) in directly proportional to the concentration of nitroimidazole within a fairly wide concentration range (upper limit $\simeq$ 10mM). Methods of analysis based on this technique have been described for the determination of metronidazole[10] and of misonidazole[11]. Unfortunately for both compounds, the overall quantity of nitroimidazole is determined, including the non-reduced metabolites present in the sample.

A detailed description of the polarographic technique and of its applications in this field of research has been discussed in the lecture by Roffia.

UV and visible spectrophotometric techniques

A quantitative treatment of the absorption of radiation energy in matter is described by the Lambert-Beer law:

$$\text{Log } \frac{I_0}{I} = A = \varepsilon_\lambda . C. d$$

I_0 = intensity of the incident becom

I = intensity of the emerging becom

ε_λ = molar extinction coefficient

C = molar concentration

d = optical path

In order for a given substance to be suitable for spectrophotometric determination, it is necessary that it absorbs in the spectral range explored (220-750 nm). In table 1 spectra data for a number of nitroimidazoles are reported[10].

TABLE 1

5, nitro-imidazole derivatives	λ_{max}	ε
nitronidazole	323 nm	9.5×10^3
DA 3837	318 "	8.8×10^3
DA 3853	332 "	6.0×10^3
DA 3831	350 "	5.3×10^3
DA 3851	332 "	1.02×10^3
DA 3821	317 "	9.08×10^3
2, nitro-imidazole derivatives		
misonidazole	324 "	7.9×10^3
LP 8711	313	9.17×10^3

In the case where the centrifuged biological fluid under investigation does not show an appreciable absorption in the spectral range covered by the absorption maximum of the drug, its concentration can be deduced directly from the spectrum, without any preliminary separation. For example, the following method has been utilized: to 0.5 ml of blood sample, extracted at different times after administration of the drug, 15,5 ml of ethanol were added in a centrifuge tube. After centrifugation of 3000 rpm for 10 min, the clear supernatant was directly analyzed in the spectrophotometer, using as blank the supernatant obtained from the blood extracted immediately prior to drug administration.

In Fig. 4 the spectrum obtained with blood taken 10 hours after administration is reported[10].

In Fig. 5 the values obtained are given as a function of time[10].

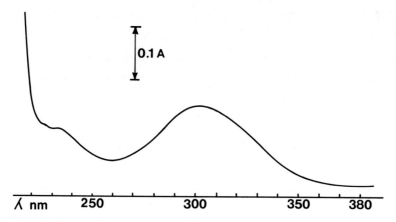

Fig. 4. Absorption spectrum of blood sample containing metronidazole.

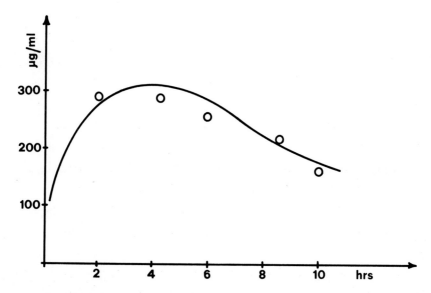

Fig. 5. Concentration of metronidazole in blood samples in a patient over a 10 hr period.

A disadvantage of this technique, as in the case with polarography, is its low selectivity with respect to the various metabolites. This can be improved by extraction with a solvent in which the drug is very soluble. This extraction must occur at controllted pH and the extraction yield must be known (otherwise, the internal standard method may by used). The method is the more selective, the lower the solubility of interferring compounds in the extracting solvent. A practical way for using this technique is a follows.

Extraction from plasma: 2 ml of plasma are treated with 6 ml H_2O and 2 ml of concentrated HCL. (The same must be done with the control plasma and with a plasma sample containing internal standard). The mixture is tirred and left at 70° on a water bath for 15-20', centrifuged for 10' at 5°C so as to obtain a clear supernatant (if the surnatant is not clear, the centrifugation must be repeated). 8 ml of supernatant are transferred to a test tube, 2 ml of phosphate buffer 1M at pH 7 are added and the solution adjusted to pH 7 with NaOH. After extracting twice with 10 ml of Ethyl Acetate, the extract is evaporated at 65°.

The residue is dissolved with a known volume of ethanol and a spectro-photometer reading is taken.

Chromatographic techniques: Chromatography techniques that are better suited (and have been employed) to the separation of the compounds with radiosensitizing properties are P.C.(paper chromatography), TLC (thin layer chrom.), GC (gaschrom.) and HPLC (high pressure liquid chromatography). The first method, which is simple and sensitive, is not sufficiently accurate for a routine analysis. The third requires some time for the extraction and derivation of the compound since radiosensitizing compounds have generally too high boiling points for gas chromatography to be directly utilizable for their analysis.

Thin layer chromatography: (TLC) In this kind of chromatography a solid support, e.g. silica gel, cellulose, alumine, polyamide is spread uniformly on a glass plate or other inert material to a thickness of 0.2 - 2 mm. The mixture to be separated is placed with a microsyringe at 1-2 cm from the rim of the plate before the plate is put into a closed chamber (developer) containing the solvent; i.e. the mobile phase. The solvent rising through capillary action elutes, with different velocities, the components of the mixture, so that separation is achieved. For each substance, a characterist parameter, which is a function of the solvent and of the experimental conditions, is defined, i.e. the ratio between the velocity with which the unknown substance and the solvent move, $Rf = \dfrac{dx}{ds}$ where dx: distance travelled by the component; ds: distance travelled by the solvent.

The various substances are detected by exposing the plate to reagents which give rise to coulored compounds or compounds which fluoresce. TLC has good resolution and sensitivity and allows the detection of as little as 10^{-9} g and is extremely useful in the field of qualitative analysis. On the other hand, it presents limitations for quantitative determinations. An example of its application is the simultaneous determination of Flagyl and misonidazole in blood. Extraction is carried out with ethyl acetate according to the method described in the spectrophotometrical section. The residue is dissolved in 100 ml ethyl acetate and quantitatively transferred to a silica gel 20x20 plate. For development over 15 cm, the solvent used is the mixture $CHCl_3$ - CH_3COOH - CH_3OH:85/10/5. The plate is examined under UV light at 254 nm and the areas are identified using standards developed together with the extracts. (Flagyl: RF=0.34, Misonidazole RF=0.48). The corresponding areas are removed and the gel is collected in centrifuge tubes. 5ml MeOH are added, stirring for 1 min and centrifuging for 5 min at 2000 rpm. The supernatants are examined spectrophotometrycally.

Also of interest is the utilization of PC and TLC in the investigation of the metabolic behaviour of drugs. In Table 2, data for separation of metronidazole from its main metabolites using PC are reported[4]. Investigation of this type however, are considerably simplified by the use of radioactive isotopes which allows a rapid identification of metabolites. This technique has been largely utilized for studying misonidazole metabolism by Flockhart et al.[7].

TABLE 2

CHROMATOGRAPHY OF METRONIDAZOLE AND ITS MAIN METABOLITES

	U.V. Light	Rf value in solvent:		
		A	B	C
1-(2-hydroxyethyl)-2-hydroxymethyl 5-nitroimidazole	Abs.	0.72	0.80	0.74
1-(2-hydroxyethyl)-5-nitroimidazole	Abs.	0.75	0.78	0.77
Metronidazole	Abs.	0.80	0.85	0.80
1-acetic acid-2-methyl-5- -nitroimidazole	Abs.	0.14	0.63	0.70

Substrate: Whatman n. 1, paper.

Solvent systems used:
  A. Butanol saturated with water,
  B. n-Propanol: Ammonia (70:30),
  C. Butanol:Acetic acid: Water (120:30:50).

High pressure liquid chromatography. This technique is relatively recent technique which is developing very rapidly and shows considerable potential. The recent improvement of liquid chromatography is due to the introduction of highly sensitive detectors of low dead-volume. The velocity, sensitivity and resolution are particularly favourable for analytical applications, and at present, this is the best analytical system for the separation of nitroimidazoles. In order to obtain high speed analysis through the use of narrow columns containing very fine grain particles high pressures must be applied to the mobile liquid phase. The efficiency of the column determines the width of the peaks and is a function of the flow velocity, the particle dimension in the stationary phase and the column diameter etc. Peak separation is determined by the selectivity of the column, i.e. by the nature of both stationary phase and mobile phase.

The efficiency of the column is expressed quantitatively through the number of theoretical plates, $N = 16 \left(\frac{tr}{W}\right)^2$ where tr is the retention of the sample and W the peak width measured at the base. N is proportional to the column height, so that it is preferable to express the efficiency with the equivalent height of a theoretical plate (HETP, or simply H),

$H = \dfrac{L}{N}$ where L is the lenght of the column.

The most common techniques used in HPCL are LSC and BPC. As far as chromatographic analysis of nitromidazoles is concerned, the most advantageous technique is BPC[*].

Bonded phase chromatography, (BPC). A large number of chemical species can be bound to absorber particles and in practice three types of chemical bounds are used when silica gel acts as support.

Chemical modification of the silica gel surface affects the retention characteristics. The greatest variations are observed when the stationary phase is made more hydrophobic through the presence of ODS[**] groups and is therefore used in the inverted phase. The compounds which are weakly retained on silica are separated in BPC. The real separation mechanism in BPC is not yet fully determined, but it appears that it can be assimilated to partition chromatography or to absroption chromatography on a non-polar stationary phase. This "Bondedphase" chromatography is of considerable advantage whenever the components are in aqueous phase, particularly in biological fluids, since the eluent, at variance with LSC, is generally a polar solvent (H_2O, acetonitrile, etc.).

Detectors

The resolution characteristics of liquid chromatography are essentially a function of the column, while its sensitivity is essentially determined by the detector. The major factors defining the performance of a detector are:

a) sensitivity (defined as the ratio between the signal generated by the detector and the sample quantity);

b) detector limit (minimum amount of sample that can be determined and which give rise to a response at least twice as high as the noise);

---

[*]   LSC = liquid solid chromatography
     BPC = bonded phase chromatography.

[**] ODS = octadecylsilane.

c) linearity;

d) response reproducibility.

For analyzing radiosensitizers which give a UV absorption spectrum, UV detectors are generally used even if, for nitroimidazoles, polarographic detectors could be employed.

Quantative analysis

The retention time is characteristic of a given compound for a given set of experimental conditions. In a good instrument, this is highly reproducible (within 2%) and this allows computerized identification of peaks.

There are essentially two ways of correlating the signal with the amount of substance producing it. Generally the peak are is used, and its measurement can be obtained in three ways: triangulation, weighing planimetry or digital integration.

Conversion of numerical data into composition

a) Normalization: the percentage of x in a mixture is expressed as % x = $=A_x f_x / \sum^n A_n . f_n$. A is the peak area and f the response factor, accounting for the different sensitivities or the detector with regard to different compounds. This method requires that all peaks are eluted.

b) Internal standard: this method eliminates injection errors, and whenever the standard is introduced before sampling, it compensates for sample preparation errors.

The internal standard must have the following requisites:

1) it must be completely resolved;

2) its retention time must be close to that of the compound examined;

3) its concentration must be similar to that of the unknown compound;

4) it must be absent in the sample under investigation.

The results are expressed as follows:

$$x = \frac{A_x f_x W_s}{A_s f_s}$$

A = peak area, f = response factor

W_s = quantity of the standard compound

s = standard

x = unknown

c) external calibration: this method utilizes the direct comparison between the area of the unknown peak and that of the peak obtained by directly injecting the standard.

Qualitative analysis

Besides being identified through its retention characteristics, a component can be identified at the column outlet by utilizing techniques commonly used in qualitative analysis. This can be done by collecting the various fractions and analyzing them successively, or a direct coupling of chromatograph and analyzer can be applied. (e.f.: HPLC - mass spectrometry).

Application of HPLC to the separation of misonidazole and metronidazole from their metabolites

The lower limit for determination of misonidazole in plasma is 5 $\mu g/ml$ [13]. Among various support materials commercially available, C_{18} bonded silica types seem to be best suited for the separation of both misonidazole and metronidazole from their respective metabolites[14,15]. Some recent work has shown that for misonidazole and its o-demethylated metabolite, an even better separation can be achieved by utilizing columns with C_{22} bonded silica[16]. This method is very well suited for the analysis of urine samples, homogenate tissue and blood plasma. A necessary preliminary operation is the deproteinization of samples. This is carried out by adding methanol and centrifugation or by passing through Amicon filters.

Deproteinization in general does not interfere with the recovery efficiency of the compound by more than 5% Table 3 reports data for chromatographic separation of misonidazole and of its leading o-demethylated metabolite and for the separation of metronidazole from its primary metabolites.

TABLE 3

SYSTEMS	RETENTION TIME
Misonidazole (RO 07-0582)	4.1 min
Misonidazole o-demethylated (RO 05-9963)	2.3 min
Column: Bondapak C_{18} (octadecylsilane)	30 cm x 3.9 mm ID
Solvent: methanole/H_2O 19/81 v/v	detector UV 313 nm
Metronidazole	5.7 min
1- Acetic acid deriv.	4.5 min
(2-hydroximethyl) deriv.	3.3 min
Column: Bondapak C_{18}	
Solvent: MeOH-CH_3CN-0.005MKH_2PO_4(pH4)	4:3:93 v/v

In Fig. 6 are reported the chromatograms obtained from methanol extracts[7] of blood plasma of a patient treated with misonidazole:

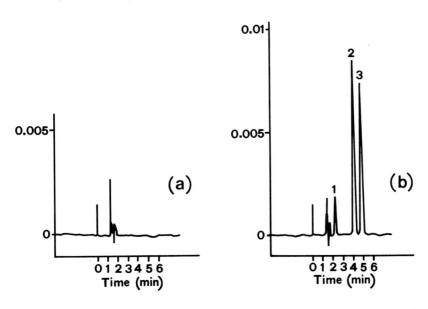

Fig. 6. Sample: a) immediately after administration; b) 2 hrs later.
1: o-demethylated metabolite; 2: misonidazole; 3: internal standard

200

a) sample taken immediately before drug administration;

b) sample taken 2 hours after oral administration of 3g m^2 of misonidazole.

Another separation by HPLC of a mixture of 2 nitro-imidazoles is shown in

Fig. 7 with a very high resolution[10].

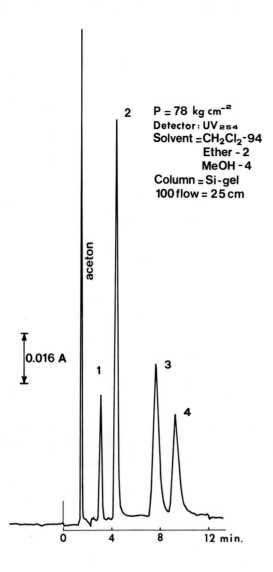

Fig. 7. Separation by HPLC of 5-nitroimidazoles: 1) 5-nitroimidazole -1,H;
2) metronidazole; 3) DA3853; 4) DA3838.

REFERENCES

1. Dische, S., Saunders, M.I., Lee, M.E., Adams, G.E., Flockhart, I.R., (1977) Br. J. Cancer, 35, 567.

2. Flockhart, I.R., Sheldon, P.W., Stratford, J.I. and Watts, M.E., (1978) Int. J. Radiat. Biol., 34, 914.

3. Adams, G.E., (1978) First lecture, this proceedings.

4. Stambaugh, J.E., Feo, L.G. and Manthei, R.W., (1967) Life Sci., 6, 1811-19.

5. Manthei, R.W. and Feo, L.G., (1964) Wiadomosci Parazytol., 2-3, 177-9.

6. Adams, G.E., Flockhart, I.R., Smithen, C.E., Stratford, I.J., Wardmann, P. and Watts, M.E., (1976) Radiat. Res., 67, 9.

7. Flockhart, I.R., Large, P., Troup, D., Malcom, S.L. and Marten, R.T., (1978) Xenobiotica, 8, 97-105.

8. Alessandri, A., Perazzi, A., Zerilli, L.F., Ferrari, P. and Martinelli, E., (1977) Drug. Metab. Disposition, 6, 109-13.

9. Cavalleri, B., Volpe, G., Arioli, V. and Lancini, G., (1977) J. Med. Chem., 20, 1522-5.

10. Gattavecchia, E. and Breccia, A., work in progress.

11. De Silva, J.A.F., Munno, N. and Strojny, N., (1970) L. Pharm.Sci., 59, 201.

12. Foster, J.L., Flockhart, I.R., Dische, S., Gray, A., Lenox-Smith, I. and Smithe, C.E., (1975) Br. J. Cancer, 31, 679.

13. Workman, P., Little, C.J., Macten, T.R., Flockhart, I.R. and Bleen, N.M., (1978) J. Chromatog., 145(3), 507-12.

14. Little, C.J., Dale, A.D. and Evans, M.B., (1978) J. Chromatog., 153(2), 381-9.

15. Wheeler, L.A., De Meo, M., Halula, M., George, L. and Heseltime, P., (1978) Antimicrob. Agents Chemoter., 13, 205-9.

16. Little, C.J., Dale, A.D. and Evans, M.B., (1978) J. Chromatog., 153(2), 543-5.

© 1979 Elsevier/North-Holland Biomedical Press
Radiosensitizers of Hypoxic Cells
A. Breccia, C. Rimondi and G.E. Adams eds.

PROBLEMS AND PROSPECTIVES OF METRONIDAZOLE IN RADIOTHERAPY

C. RIMONDI

Dept. of Radiation Therapy Malpighi Hospital, Bologna, Italy

INTRODUCTION

The results of radiation therapy, e.g. for carcinoma of the uterine cervix
(one of the most commonly-treated neoplastic sites) for local control and
5 years' survival (Marcial, 1977)[1] show that successful results are most
favourable in the early stages of the disease, but are modest in the advanced
stages. Even in the early stages unsuccessful results are not uncommon at all.
The existence of cells that are chronically hypoxic and hence radioresistant,
is considered to be the most important cause of failure of radiation therapy.
This is because this sub-population of cells (whose proportion changes from
tumour to tumour) cannot be eradicated by radiation treatment and it can be
responsible for further growth of the neoplasm even when all the well-oxygenated
cells have been killed by radiation. In particular, different proportions of
hypoxic cells can influence considerably the dose of radiation needed to
obtain local control of the tumours. Thus for some large tumours where the
proportion of these cells may be very high, the dose needed may be higher than
that tolerated by healthy tissues (Figs. 1-2).

The electron-affinic hypoxic cell radiosensitizers offer a good
possibility of acting specifically, both indirectly as radiosensitizers and
directly for their cytotoxicity on this subpopulation, without increasing
the damaging effect of radiation on the cellular elements of peripheral
healthy tissues as they are well-oxygenated.

1. CHARACTERISTICS OF METRONIDAZOLE

Of the nitroderivatives, a 5-nitroimidazole, metronidazole (Flagyl) has
been the first to be used as a radiosensitizer, particularly because of its
low toxicity.

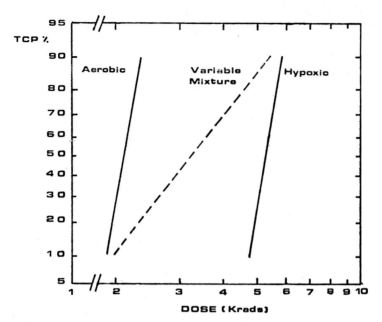

Fig. 1. Theoretical tumour cure probability curves based on the results of animal tumour studies for homogeneously aerobic or hypoxic tumours, and for a series of tumours in wich the proportion of hypoxic cells was variable. The shallow slope of this latter (variable-mixture) curve reflects a wide range of probabilities for cure of individual tumours in a series in which hypoxia may vary from complete to non-existent. (Fletcher G.H., 1973)[2].

Metronidazole is a well known drug utilized in the treatment of trichomoniasis in doses of 1-2 gm daily without particular problems of tolerance, except in the rare cases of haemolytic crisis due to a lack of the enzyme glucose-6-phosphate dehydrogenase. This drug was shown by Asquith, et al. (1973)[3], to radiosensitize hypoxic cells *in vitro* and *in vivo*.

Radiosensitization has been seen both in hypoxic skin and in solid tumours in the mouse. More recently, this drug has been shown to possess direct cytotoxic properties against hypoxic cells *in vitro*. The mechanism of this effect is independent of the mechanism of radiation sensitization. The cytocidal activity of metronidazole on anaerobic microorganisms but not on aerobic microorganisms has been previously observed. The activity depends on the concentration of the drug and on the duration of contact but is

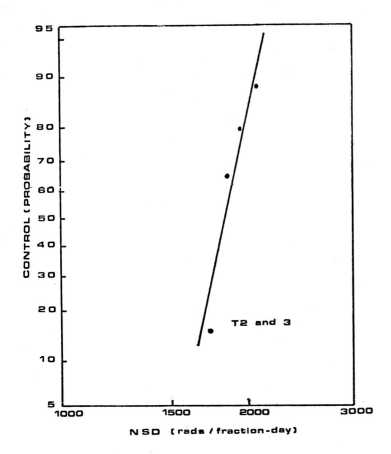

Fig. 2. Graphs of probability of control versus NSD (Fletcher G.H., 1973)[2].

present only in hypoxic cells. Because of this property it is believed by
some authors that this drug may have independent application in the chemotherapy
of tumours with specific activity against hypoxic cells (Mohindra J.,
Rauth A.M., 1976)[4].

2. ACTIVITY OF METRONIDAZOLE AT THE CELLULAR LEVEL AND ON TUMOURS IN EXPERIMENTAL ANIMALS

The radiosensitizing effect of this drug has been demonstrated at the
cellular level where D_o was reduced to 243 rads through addition of 1 mg/g of

metronidazole to cultures *in vitro* of the EMT 6 tumour, compared with 446 rads without sensitizer (Brown, 1975)[5]. *In vivo*, in tumours transplanted into C3H mice, the TCD_{50} was 3100 rads after administration of 1 mg/g of Metronidazole 30 minutes before irradiation with a single dose, and 4041 rads without radiosensitizer, giving an E.R. of 1,3 ± 0,6 (Begg, 1974)[6].

In a series of experiments on several experimental tumours in mice using different end-points including re-growth delay, etc., the ER for metronidazole in doses of 1 mg/g was 1,3-2,1 (that of misonidazole in the same doses (1,6-2,9). (C.R.O.S., 1976)[7].

In fractionated irradiation given in 5 daily sessions, with administration of 0,1 mg/g of Flagyl intra-peritoneally 10 minutes before each radiation treatment, the E.R. was reduced to 1,13 in comparison with 1,20 for the same dose in a single irradiation (Stone, 1976)[8].

3. RADIOSENSITIZATION IN MAN

The evaluation in quantitative terms of sensitization which is generally expressed as a percentage of the oxygen effect or as DMF, is very difficult in man and almost impossible at a clinical-therapeutic level. Data from studies *in vitro* and *in vivo* e.g. in tumours of experimental animals which vary from one system to another can only indicate approximate values in man. For example, the metabolism of drugs in animals may differ the human one.

There is a good correlation between the sensitiziting effects and drug concentration in the medium or in blood, both for data *in vitro* (ADAMS)[9], and for sensitization of hypoxic skin in man (DISCHE) (Fig. 3)[10].

For the levels of metronidazole attainable in man, the effect of sensitization is estimated at 10-20% (Urtasun et al.[11], 1975, Deutsch, 1975)[12].

4. TOXICOLOGY AND PHARMACO-KINETIC RESEARCH (Phase I)

Phase I of research of this drug in man concerns the kinetic characteristics and the toxicology after repeated administration. These data are necessary for determining a fractionated radiation treatment.

The research of Urtasun et al.[11], largely coincides with our study. They have demonstrated the following data:

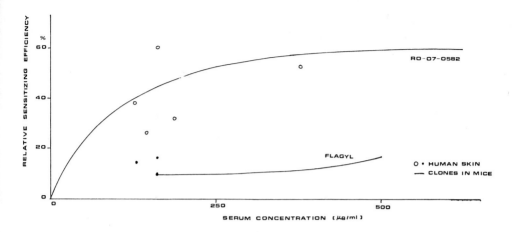

Fig. 3. The sensitizing effect of Flagyl and Ro 07-0582, expressed as a percentage of that which can be achieved by 100% oxygen, on artificially hypoxic skin, as a function of serum concentration for mice and men. The human data correspond to the curves obtained from mice[13].

- For doses of 2,5 gm/m^2, the maximum concentration in the blood is 70-80 μg/ml and is reached after approximately four hours.
- Intermediate doses of 4 gm/m^2 which were those most commonly utilized in our study, show a maximum concentration in the blood of 110-180 μg/ml after two hours, decreasing slightly after four hours, Fig. 4.
- The drug is very stable with a long half life of 10-12 hours. It is not metabolized and is eliminated slowly with almost complete elimination after 48 hours.
- The major problem is gastric tolerance, with nausea and sometimes vomiting generally appearing rather late in the treatment. This, therefore, does not appear to interfere with the absorption of the drug. After a prolonged treatment a marked anorexia may appear.

Urtasun et al.[14] have demonstrated that the drug crosses the blood-brain barrier and its concentration in the liquor approaches that in the blood.

The Canadian authors[14] have further demonstrated that the concentrations reached at the tumour site are only slightly inferior to those in blood. These concentration are reached at the centre of the tumour with a delay of

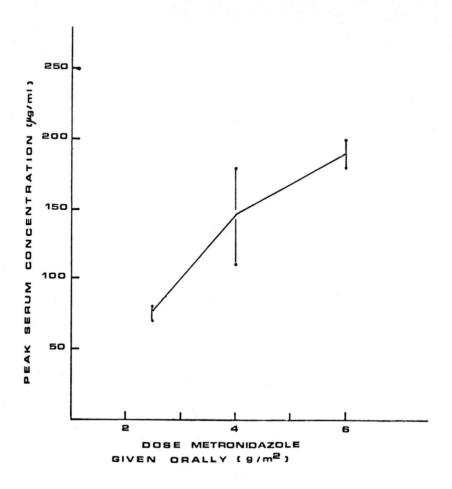

Fig. 4. Serum concentration of Metronidazole (ug/ml) as a function of dose given orally (g/m²).

approximately 30 minutes with respect to the maximum blood concentration. This study was carried out on biopsied material obtained from superficial metastatic tumours.

No disorders were noted in the blood or in the principle excretory organs following single or multiple administration. These were checked immediately after administration and up to 12-18 months later. These observations coincided with those seen in our patients.

5. GENERAL DRUG TOLERANCE

In fact, especially for pelvic treatment, the problem of gastric tolerance
is important and cannot be totally controlled by the use of antiemetic drugs,
as suggested by Urtasun et al.[11]. This problem may be severe enough to
necessitate the suspension of this medication. The low gastric tolerance
may be due in part to the administration of the large number of tablets
(30-40) necessary to reach the suggested dose. Gastric disturbances, however,
remain even for the special preparations (tablets of 1 gm) which allow the
total number of tablets to be reduced to 7-11.

6. PRELIMINARY CLINICAL EXPERIENCE WITH METRONIDAZOLE

In relation to the toxicity of the drug it has been found opportune to
modify the fractionation scheme of 200 rads per day and 1,000 rads per week.
For example, Urtasun et al.[11] utilized a fractionation scheme with a higher
single dose (330-480 rads) 2-3 times a week for three weeks.

In patients afflicted with bronchial carcinoma and with supratentorial
glioblastoma, 6 g/m^2 of metronidazole have been administered 4 hours before
every session of radiotherapy No undesirable reaction, immediate or after
a short time, have been noticed in skin, (including subcutaneous tissues),spinal
cord, lung, or for the appearance of alopecia and regrowth of hair.

Karim (1977)[15] has used metronidazole in the treatment of 48 patients
with cervical and gastro-intestinal (G.I.) tumours in advanced stages. He
administrered daily doses of 2.5 gm for 5 days a week for a total treatment
time of 5-7 weeks. This dose was well tolerated without toxic signs in
the blood, excretory organs and the nervous system. The total dose received
was 6,000-7,600 rads in the cervical region with regression of the tumour
in 10 of 23 patients (43%). 5,500 rads were used in 8 patients with carcinoma
of the GI tract with a positive response in four cases. It can be concluded
that even the modest sensitization, due to the low dose of Metronidazole used,
resulted in a higher than normal local tumour control.

7. CLINICAL EXPERIENCE WITH METRONIDAZOLE AND RADIOTHERAPY WITH MULTIPLE DAILY SESSIONS

We used in our patients, multiple daily treatment according to the scheme proposed by Littbrand and Backstrom, because of our past experience with this method which has the advantage of exploiting the persistence of high concentration of the drug in circulation[16]. We administered the drug on alternate days at a dose of 4 gm/m^2, irradiating at intervals of 2-6-10 hours after administration, thus delivering a focal dose of 100 rads per treatment. On the intermediate days the radiation treatment is carried out in the same manner. The duration of the treatment is three weeks.

We treated ten patients by this method. Daily doses of 6.5-7 gm were administered each other day for a total dose of 57 to 63 gm in three weeks. There was good general tolerance except for nausea and some episodes of vomiting. The radiation treatment was carried out by means of cobalt therapy using the technique of fixed fields. These fields of irradiation were adjusted so as to adequately encompass the tumour mass. Multiple daily treatments of 100 rads to the focus were used. These were separated by four hours according to the method already proposed by Littbrand and utilized by us for the treatment of numerous patients.

According to polarographic determinations, the maximum concentration in the blood was reached within two hours after administration. These values then reduced slowly and progressively to 50% of the initial concentrations at a time of 10-12 hours after administration (Fig. 5)[17].

Based on these data, the first radiation treatment is given two hours after medication and successively after the 6th and 10th hours.

The treatment was carried out in patients affected by carcinomas of various locations in advanced stages or metastatic disease with limited survival time in which it was impossible to achieve definite results with the usual therapy.

Haematogically, the treatment was well tolerated. The most common metabolic variables (glycemia, proteinemia, creatininemia, bilirubinemia, etc.) measured during the treatment and continously up to four months after the end of the

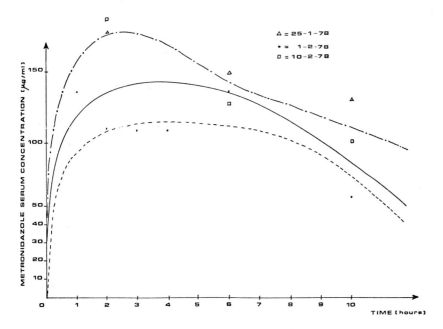

Fig. 5. Serum concentration of Metronidazole at different times following oral administration of 4 g/m^2 in three different days[17].

treatment show significant changes.

Except in one case of transitory hallucinations, a type of microzoopsia, no important neurological alterations were revealed. Reactions of the skin and of the mucous tissue;appeared generally at the end of the cycle of treatment and their duration and regression did not vary from that normally seen.

Objective regressions of the tumours mass completely or above 50% were observed in 6 out of 10 patients treated while 4 failed to respond or responded insignificantly. In these 10 patients the clinical observations may be summarised as below:

The cutaneous and mucosal reactions included in the irradiated area, both immediately and after a certain period of time, do not appear to be significantly altered with respect to those observed with the same method of fractionation and technique of irradiation. Also the appearance of pelvic fibrosis in three cases followed for a longer period of time did not present extension or morphological characteristics different from those normally observed.

8. PHASE II - METRONIDAZOLE CLINICAL RESEARCH

In subsequent clinical phase II studies Urtasun, et al.[14], utilized Metronidazole in a group of randomized patients. These patients had a supratentorial glioblastoma and were divided into two groups.

The first group (15 patients) was treated with only radiation therapy. The second group (16 patients) was given 6 gm/m^2 of metronidazole, followed after four hours by radiation therapy.

The graphs of survival rates according to a Kaplan-Meier fit (Fig. 6)

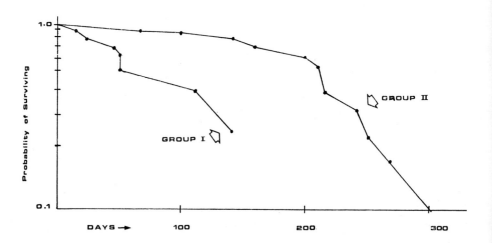

Fig. 6. KAPLAN-MEIER Survival plots showing the probability of surviving past time t for patients in Group I (radiation alone - 15 Pts) and in Group II (radiation combined with Metronidazole - 16 Pts)[14].

show a difference which is statistically significant at the level of 0.02 according to the test of Wilcoxan-Gehan. The two curves shown are analogous except that one can observe a displacement of 4.5 months before tumour reccurrence and subsequent death in the patients treated with radiation therapy and Metronidazole, both in the actuarial curve and in the final curve when all the patients had died.

The objection has been raised against this trial that the control group was not treated with optimal fractionation and total dosage. This clinical trial was therefore repeated in four randomized groups of patients with supertentorial glioblastomas:

1st group of controls was treated with conventional dose and fractionation;

2nd group was treated with Metronidazole (6 gm/m^2) plus radiotherapy (elevated dose of radiation 430 rads on alternate days for three weeks);

3rd group was treated with Metronidazole (6 mg/m^2) administered after radiation therapy to assay its eventual direct cytotoxic action;

4th group treated as the 2nd group but utilizing Misonidazole (1-1.5 gm/m^2) in place of Metronidazole.

9. CRITICAL EVALUATION OF DRUGS NON AVAILABLE

The ideal characteristics for clinical use of a radiosensitizing drug would be the following:

1 - Therapeutic dose much less than the toxic dose

2 - An large distribution of the drug

3 - Capacity of the drug to diffuse to reasonable distances in a non-
-vascularized cell mass (greater than 200 μm), in order to reach all
the hypoxic cells

4 - Stability of the drug, which must not be rapidly metabolized or eliminated

5 - It must be effective during the entire cellular cycle, or at least in
the initial phases of the cycle, since it is probable that hypoxic cells
are arrested in this stage

6 - It must be effective at the relatively low doses of radiation used
in fractionated radiotherapy.

Neither of the two drugs actually available show all of these characteristics, in fact Metronidazole has only a modest radiosensitizing effectiveness and therefore must be administered at relatively high doses. The toxicity is modest,but gastric tolerance, at least in our experience, is often low with notable tendency to vomiting. This may be in part due to the location of the tumors which we treated most frequently (gynelogical, bladder and rectum cancer).

The administration of metronidazole for three weeks has induced in some patients marked anorexia which regresses following the end of treatment.

Misonidazole has a higher radiosensitizing efficiency but is, however, highly neurotoxic at higher doses and therefore proposed dosages were significantly reduced as reported by Dr. Dische[18].

Furthermore, except for the lower dosages of 2,5 gm, the use of these drugs has required a modification of the common scheme of fractionation of the dose and of the total doses with possible consequences in the effectiveness and tolerance of the treatment which are difficult to evaluate.

These modifications of the schemes of fractionation which are acceptable in palliative treatment of advanced tumours, raise problems in treatment with radical curative possibilities and must not be applied outside of a clinically controlled and randomized study.

Based on the above data one will be faced with the problem of the selection of the drug when they are equally available. The minor effectiveness of Metronidazole with respect to Misonidazole may be compensated by better tolerance and with the possibility of administering 5-7 time superior doses, for which, at least to day in the laboratory experiments, the radiosensitizing effects obtainable is not very different for the two drugs.

As it has been said, the doses of radiosensitizer permissible in man are much less than those used in the laboratory experiments. Also the doses of radiation used in a clinical field are significanty less than those often used in animals.

It therefore appears that a compromise is required also in the clinical field, between the dose of radiosensitizer and the dose of radiation. It can be asked; if with the dose of radiosensitizer utilizable and with the dose of radiation of radiotherapy is it still possible to demonstrate the effectiveness of this combination? An attempt at a quantitative evaluation of the optimal relationship between doses of the radiosensitizing drug and the dose of radiation raises notable difficulties. In fact, in addition to the problem of calculating the electron concentration that is produced in the tumours due to the irradiation, and of the molecules of radiosensitizer present in the same area, the distribution of the drug must be evaluated, particularly in the hypoxic regions.

10. PROBLEMS OF DOSE FRACTIONATION IN RADIOTHERAPY WITH RADIOSENSITIZERS

The use of radiosensitizing drugs proposes a series of problems involving the fractionation of the dose which have been resolved in various situations (Dische, et al., 1976)[18].

- The use of relatively modest doses of Metronidazole (2.5 gm) daily with normal fractionation and total irradiation dose (5,000-6,000 rads in 5-7 week) (Karim)[15]

- Reduction of the number of treatments spaced in time (9 fractions in three weeks) with high doses of Metronidazole (6 gm/m^2) (Urtasun)[14]

- Administration of the radiosensitizer with only some of the radiation therapy treatments (3 gm of Misonidazole once a week for four weeks) (Wiltshire, et al., 1977)[19]

- Combinations with multiple daily treatments to exploit the long half-life of the drug.

As treatment of choice we have selected the latter, which presents both advantages and disadvantages.

- The effect of sensitization of Metronidazole must be added to that due to the multiple daily fractionation

- The simple doses of 100 rads are actually rather low and it must be asked if they are the most useful to identify the likely effect of sensitization produced by the drug.

A definitive choice of the most advantagenous combination may be derived from a series of clinically controlled trials.

CONCLUSIONS:

The radiosensitizing drugs, could be used in future as adjuvants to radiotherapy, in those cases where radiotherapy alone offers a poor prognosis for local control of neoplastic disease, even when radiotherapy is used with the best technical methods and according to a rational scheme of fractionation.

As an aid for the development of RT, experiments with these drugs presents rather interesting possibilities:

- the sensitization seems to be effective only on neoplastic tissues, in particular in its hypoxic component and not in healthy well-oxygenated tissues. This gives therefore, an increase in the therapeutic index.
- The effectiveness of the drugs and the doses actually used are still not optimal, especially if compared with the O_2 effect. We must instead ask ourselves what is the effect obtainable from sensitization by 10-20% wheter that can be translated into demonstrable benefits at the clinical level.
- In particular, one may have difficulty based on the fact that use of a radiosensitizing drug may necessitate a modification of the optimal fractionation.
- An additional factor is the importance of fractionation in influencing reoxygenation of the surviving hypoxic cells. It is probable that sensitizers with those schemes of dose fractionation which are truly optimal and lead to efficient reoxygenation, can add little and some of the advantages may be lost. However, advantages may still be obtained in cases where the fractionation is not ideal, or when the reoxygenation cannot occur in an effective way.
- Possibility of acquiring further information, particularly in human neoplastic pathology, on the importance of hypoxic cells, also in respect of the evolution of the tumour.
- The prospect of beginning new researches on more effective and less toxic approaches to other adjuvant therapy of RT.
- Complementary surgical operation for tumours with an incomplete response which are susceptable to exeresis, may be facilitated if the effectiveness of the treatment is increased, or the dose can be reduced while still giving a higher effectiveness. With these methods, one is further able to acquire useful material for anatomical and histopathological studies of the eventual modification of tumours following use of sensitizers.
- Chemotherapy as an adjuvant for the prevention of metastasis has a more effective result if the local and regional results of the radiation treatment have been improved by treatment combined with radiosensitizers.

- The association of radiosensitizer in post-operative radiotheraphy may be
  equally advantageous if useful concentrations of the drug could be obtained,
  at the level of intervention scar: this because of the fact that the main
  cause of failure may be due precisely to the presence of hypoxic tumour
  cells in poorly-vascularized scar tissue.

  It is of value to note the possibility of association of RT with antiblastic
  chemotherapy, particularly with those drugs for which a radiosensitizing
  effect has been postulated, even though the problems may be difficult to
  study.

The theoretical bases of Radiotherapy combined with radiosensitizers and
with chemotherapy are different:

- with radiation sensitizers, the purpose is the enhanced killing of a
  radiation-resistant subpopulation of hypoxic cells;
- with chemotherapy, the purpose is to kill all tumour cells in the short
  period of contact with the drug. In order to get a good result from
  combined therapy, the effect may be useful on by whether the eliminated cells
  could not be killed by the following radiation dose;
- the introduction of radiosensitizers has shown difficulties concerning
  time, dose, fractionation, factors that must be considered in programming
  integrated treatments;
- also for the hypoxic cell radiosensitizing drugs, the possibility of an
  antiblastc effect and direct cytotoxic action has been proposed as
  previously mentioned. Foster[20] has proposed the administration of the drug
  before beginning RT in order to eliminate or reduce the component of hypoxic
  cells. Urtasun has administrered the drug following a single RT treatment,
  despite the apparent contradiction that, due to the persistence of the drug
  in circulation, any direct cytotoxic action would add to the radiosensitizing
  effect even if the drug were administrered before irradiation.

Considering adjunctive therapy, we can make some comparisons between the use
of radiosensitizers and cytostatic agents:

- indications for therapy with radiosensitizers are those tumours where
  there is a tendency for local relapse and where the main cause of failure,
  and hence death of the patients, is the unsuccessful local cure of the

disease (e.g. carcinoma of the head, neck, soft tissue , carcinoma of the
uterus, of the bladder, cerebral neoplasm, etc.);
- the indications for adjunctive therapy with cytostatic agents refer
mostly to neoplastic lesions with high frequency of distant metastasis
(breast and lung carcinoma); another indication of therapy with
radiosensitizers (even if aimed only at improving results of palliative
treatment) concerns locally advanced tumours which are not susceptible to
surgical therapy, where an improvement of local control may prolong and
improve survival or the quality of life.

To be able to evaluate the effectiveness and the toxicology of drugs,
it is necessary to measure the concentration of the drug in the blood and
if possible also in the tumour. It is also important to determine the
maximum concentration, the time necessary to reach this concentration
and the half-life. This is necessary in order to establish the optimal
time for carrying out radiotherapy and to interpret treatment response
and any toxic effects.

ACKNOWLEDGEMENTS

I thank the editors of British J. of Radiology for fig. 1,2; International
J. of Radiation Oncology, Biology and Physics for fig. 3; an N. Engl.
J. Med. for fig. 6.

REFERENCES

1. Marcial, V.A. (1977) Carcinoma of the cervix. Present status and future
   Cancer, 39, 945-958.

2. Fletcher, G.H. (1973) Brit. J. of Radiology, 46, 1-12.

3. Asquith, J.C., Foster, J.L., Willson, R.L., Ings, R. and McFadzean, J.A.,
   (1974) Br. J. Radiol. 47, 474.

4. Mohindra, J. and Rauth, A.M. (1976) Cancer, Res., 36, 930-936.

5. Brown, J.M. (1975) Selective radiosensitization of the hypoxic cell of
   mouse tumours with the nitroimidazole, metronidazole and Ro-07-0582,
   Radiat. Res., 64, 633.

6. Begg, A.C. and Fowler, J.F. (1974) A rapid method for the determination
   of tumour RBE, Br. J. Radiol., 47, 237.

7. C.R.O.S. (1976) Radiation sensitizers, Cancer, Suppl. 37/4.

8. Stone, H.B. (1976) Int. J. Radiation Oncology, Biol., Phys., 1, 1133-1137.

9. Dische, S. (1978) Int. Jour. Rad. Oncology, Biol., Phys., 4, 157-170.

10. Adams, G.E. (1974) Proc. 11th Int. Cancer Congres, Florence, Excerpta Medica.

11. Urtasun, R.C., Chapman, J.D., Band, P., Rabin, H.R., Fryer, C.G. and Sturmwind, J. (1975) Radiology 177, 129, 133.

12. Deutsch, G., Foster, J.L., Mc Fadzean, J.A. and Parnell, M. (1975) Brit. J. Cancer, 31, 75-80.

13. Denekamp, J. and Fowler, J.F. (1978) Int. Jour. Rad. Oncology, Biol., Phys., 4, 146.

14. Urtasun, R.C., Miller, J.D.R., Frunchak, V., Koziol, D., Band, P.R., Chapman, J.D. and Feldstein, M.L. (1977) Brit. J. Radiology, 50, 603-604.

15. Karim, A.B.M.F., (1977) Response of advanced tumours to Metronidazole: a pilot study
Abstracts of paers presented at the 8th L.H. Gray Conference.

16. Rimondi, C. and Busutti, L. (1978) Atti XII Congr. Naz. AIRBM Roma 1977, EMSI.

17. Breccia, A., Rimondi, C. and Busutti, L. (1978) L'impiego di farmaci RSCI in radioterapia. Lezione di aggiornamento al XXVIII Congr. Nazion. Ass. It. rad. med. e Med. nucl., Rimini.

18. Dische, S., Gray, A.J. and Zanelli, G.D. (1976) Clinical Radiology, 27, 159-166.

19. Wiltshire, C.R., Workman, P., Watson, J.V. and Bleehan, N.M. (1977) Clinical Studies with Misonidazole Abstracts of paper presented at the 8th L.H. Gray Conference.

20. Foster, J.L. (1978) Int. Journ. Rad. Oncology Biol. Phys., 4, 153-156.

CLINICAL EXPERIENCE WITH MISONIDAZOLE

STANLEY DISCHE

Marie Curie Research Wing for Oncology, Regional Radiotherapy Centre,

Mount Vernon Hospital, Northwood, Middlesex, England

ABSTRACT

The laboratory studies give promise that the hypoxic cell radiosensitizer, misonidazole, may give improved results in clinical radiotherapy.

The initial clinical work has shown that it is well absorbed when given orally; it freely diffuses into tumours; it does sensitize hypoxic cells in man as in animals and in patients with multiple deposits of tumour increased response can be seen in those nodules irradiated with misonidazole.

Neurotoxicity does limit the amount which can be given. It has now been shown that a total of 12g per square metre of surface area given over a period of at least 17 days is a safe one provided that some monitoring of serum concentration is made.

Controlled clinical trials involving many centres are now underway in many countries. The tumours under study include glioblastomas, carcinoma of cervix and head and neck tumours.

INTRODUCTION

Chemical hypoxic cell sensitizers give real hope of advance in the treatment of cancer by radiotherapy. We look forward to more cures and better palliation. As a result of much laboratory experiment misonidazole has come to the clinic as the first drug which might fulfil these expectations. By this time over 400 patients have received this drug in England, Canada, Austria, South Africa, the United States and now in France and other countries.

We now know that the drug is readily absorbed and diffuses deeply into tissue: in many clinical studies it is now quite clear that radiosensitizing concentrations can regularly be achieved in tumours. Biopsies usually reveal between 60 and 100% of the serum concentration within the tumour. In Figure 1 we can see a core taken through a carcinoma of the breast.

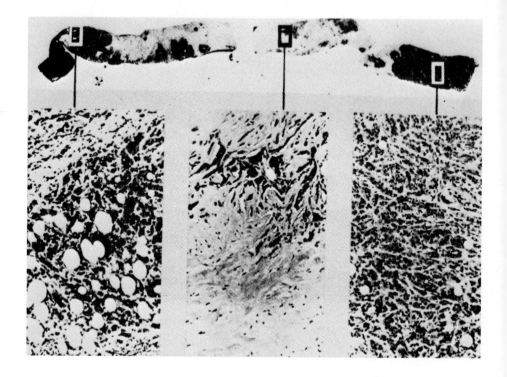

Fig. 1. (see text)

Although at the very edge of tumour there is a high concentration of fully viable tumour cells, these become fewer within the depths of the tumour and cells only seem to survive around blood vessels. A tumour such as this can be expected to have a high concentration of hypoxic cells. The central section of the core was submitted to analysis for misonidazole concentration. The level was, in fact, 99% of that in the serum at the time of biopsy.

In order to determine if hypoxic cells could be made sensitive in man we irradiated the skin of a group of patients using a radium strontium plaque. We did this under oxic and hypoxic conditions in order to see whether the drug could restore radiosensitivity. We used a complex system to make the skin hypoxic. An Esmarch's bandage was wound round the limb; a sphygmomanometer cuff applied at high pressure and then after uncoiling the Esmarch's bandage the limb was encircled in a bag of nitrogen. Under hypoxia with this system usually double the dose of radiation is required in order to achieve the same degree of pigmentation after treatment as that achieved when radiation is given under normal oxic conditions. Using hypoxia and the radiosensitizing drug, however, much enhanced reaction was achieved. As an example, in one patient after misonidazole was given 1600 rad given under hypoxic conditions gave similar pigmentation as when 800 rad were given under oxic conditions. We reduced our dose in hypoxia to 1200 rad and even then the response was greater than when 1600 rad were given under hypoxic conditions. In this case, therefore, the radiosensitivity of hypoxic skin had been taken more than halfway back to that of oxic skin by the addition of the radiosensitizing drug. (Dische, et al. 1977[1]). There was no significant alteration in the response of oxic skin.

The relative sensitizing efficiency is a measure, expressed as a percentage, of the restoration of the sensitivity of the hypoxic cells to that of those under oxic conditions. In the six patients given misonidazole, in a range of doses, the efficiencies extended from 27 to 71%. These values can be compared to 11-14% in three patients given metronidazole.

A further study was made to determine any difference in response of tumours in patients with multiple measurable metastases (Thomlinson, et al. 1976[2]) Seven patients, all of whom gave their informed consent, took part in the investigation, but three died before results were obtained. Since ionising radiation produces its predominant effect by destroying the reproductive integrity of cells and a sensitizer of hypoxic cells may be expected to reduce the number surviving, the investigation was based on observation of regrowth of similar tumours differently treated in each patient.

The most striking result came from a young woman with multiple sub-cutaneous metastases from a carcinoma of cervix. Measurement of two groups each of seven nodules with a mean diameter of 12.6 mm showed a significant difference ($P=0.05$) of the time of regrowth after single doses of 960 rad and 1120 rad, giving a measure of the discriminatory sensitivity of the system used. The re-growth seen in a third group of seven nodules treated with the lower radiation dose of 800 rad combined with a dose of misonidazole was similar to that after 960 rad alone, indicating a dose enhancement factor of 1.2.

In a second patient with metastasis in the lung from primary carcinoma of the breast, no enhancement was found; in a third there was fairly clear evidence of an enhancement though this did not reach significance in the period of survival of the patient. In a fourth a margin of improvement was seen.

Let us consider the ways in which the drug can be used with radiotherapy. There are, unfortunately, toxic effects which limit the total dose which can be given and these are discussed in another chapter.

A dose of 12g per square metre of surface area is now generally accepted as the safe minimum when misonidazole is given over a period of at least 17 days. This amount of drug can be given in different patterns. How should we administer this dose? The bulk of radiobiological evidence suggests that the greatest effect would be achieved in hypoxic cells when the highest dose of sensitizer is combined with the highest radiation dose. With a single treatment as for palliation, the sensitizer would certainly improve the response. When we move to the multi-fraction techniques used in radiotherapy for cure there are many possible patterns of administration of misonidazole. First it can be given in a few large doses each combined with a high radiation dose. A regime where six treatments with misonidazole and radiotherapy are given twice weekly over a three week period has been used by ourselves and by Sealy in Capetown (Sealy, 1978[3]).

Schemes of radiotherapy where multiple doses are given in one day may be combined with administration of misonidazole so that two or more treatments may be given by radiotherapy with just one dose of misonidazole taking advantage of the relatively long half-life of the drug.

Another approach is to give the drug once or twice a week when daily radiotherapy is employed. In this situation when the misonidazole is given the radiation dose is commonly higher than on the other occasions in the week when the radiation is given alone.

Finally, the drug can be given with a normal daily fractionated course of radiotherapy over four, five or six weeks with misonidazole being given in small doses on each occasion.

The first two techniques recognise the suggested advantage of high radiation dose and high sensitizer concentration. We must carefully examine the suggestion that small daily doses of misonidazole may also be helpful. We know that the relationship between sensitization and dose is not linear. There is a steep rise at low concentrations of sensitizer and with further increase there is a lessening benefit. (Figure 2)

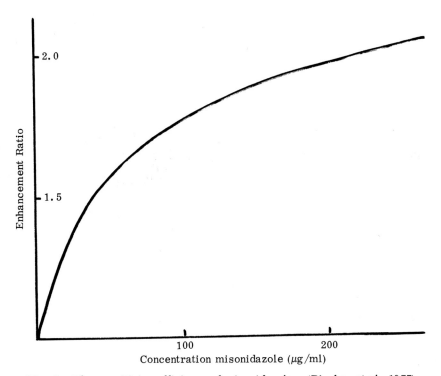

Fig. 2. The sensitizing efficiency of misonidazole. (Dische, et al. 1977)

When six doses of misonidazole are given using the permitted maximum total dose of 12 g per square metre of surface area serum concentrations of the order of 70 μg/ml are obtained. Such levels can be associated with an enhancement ratio of 1.6 to 1.7 for hypoxic cells. If daily doses are employed combined with 20 to 30 treatments by radiotherapy, serum concentrations between 18 and 26 μg/ml are normally obtained and therefore enhancement ratios of 1.3 to 1.4 can be expected for hypoxic cells. Despite the breakdown of the dose into much smaller amounts the enhancement ratio has only been halved.

When we look at the survival curves for oxic and hypoxic cells we can see that the curves tend to come together at the 150-200 rad depth dose level. Applying the known biological data, therefore, it may be that no sensitization is achieved and, in fact, there might be reduced cell kill. It is, however, extremely difficult for our biological colleagues to assess the oxygen effect at this low level of dose. We now have important data for humans in the results of the Medical Research Council's hyperbaric oxygen trials (Watson, et al. 1978[4]; Dische, 1978[5]) Of the cases treated for carcinoma of cervix, 75% were treated at Glasgow and Mount Vernon where doses were around the 200 rad per day level. There was a highly significant increase in local control level thus showing the oxygen effect is relevant at this dose level which is the common one employed in daily fractionated radiotherapy.

Finally there is the independent cytotoxic effect of the nitroimidazoles. It remains to be seen whether at the level of dose of misonidazole possible in man this effect is to be an important one, but if it is then because of the importance of the duration of exposure, daily administration of misonidazole may lead to the greatest cell-kill. We need careful biological experiments in man to increase our knowledge.

It is important that we explore all the possibilities in the combination of misonidazole with radiotherapy. However, we must be careful not to have too many trials and too many regimes when none may be adequately tested. Collaboration between Radiotherapy Centres is essential if we are to learn the value of the drug at the earliest possible time.

Is there any evidence at this early stage that misonidazole is leading to improvement in local cure rates? We have now administered the drug to over 130 patients and all of us using the drug have a favourable impression but we know that experience is fallacious and judgement difficult - we can only rely on the hard evidence of randomized controlled clinical trials. We are certainly convinced that early reactions in normal tissues are exactly as those which occur without use of the drug. In terms of tumour control we have the evidence from the use of metronidazole by Dr. Urtasun in Edmonton (Urtasun, et al. 1976[6]) where benefit in terms of prolongation of survival was shown in the treatment of glioblastoma using metronidazole. This certainly encourages us to look for even greater benefit from misonidazole known to be a much more potent agent in laboratory work.

We at Mount Vernon have shown in our hyperbaric oxygen trials in carcinoma of cervix that there is a significant correlation between the regression at the end of treatment and the long-term control. We noted a significant improvement in the immediate response of tumour observed at the end of treatment and so were able to predict the benefit seen in later follow up (Dische, 1974[7]). In our first eight patients with advanced carcinoma of cervix treated with radiotherapy and misonidazole all have shown a complete regression at the end of treatment. This is, of course, only a hint of promise and we are now pursuing a randomized controlled clinical trial.

At this time many randomized controlled clinical trials are underway or are in an advanced planning stage. In glioblastoma grades III and IV trials are underway at Cambridge, Edmonton, Alberta and Vienna. These employ a limited number of treatments combined with misonidazole. A multi-centre trial in the United Kingdom is soon to be started in England where over 20 centres will give the drug with all 20 fractions of radiotherapy. A similar trial using 30 fractions has been planned in West Germany and another by the EORTC where misonidazole is to be given with daily radiotherapy in the first three weeks of treatment.

In Capetown Professor Sealy is treating advanced oral cancer using six fractions of radiotherapy with and without misonidazole. In the United Kingdom multi-centre studies in head and neck cancer using 10 and up to 30 fractions are planned. In the United States protocols making one or more administrations of misonidazole are in phase II study in head and neck tumours as in many other sites of tumour.

In carcinoma of cervix stage III a multi-centre trial is planned in the United Kingdom where whole pelvis irradiation is followed by intra-cavitary treatment. All being given with or without misonidazole. This may be extended to become a European study. A trial in carcinoma of the bronchus using six fractions of radiotherapy with and without misonidazole has been underway at Mount Vernon since January 1977. Many other sites of tumour including oesophagus, stomach, large bowel, bladder and pancreas are being considered for study at this time. The initial exploration of the use of misonidazole with cytotoxic chemotherapeutic agents has begun and there are, of course, great possibilities there.

Hypoxic cell sensitizers have now arrived in clinical radiotherapy and oncology. It is up to clinicians to pursue their study with scientific purpose and in collaborative randomized controlled clinical trials to determine whether the first of the agents to arrive with us in the clinic is going to be of benefit to our patients.

REFERENCES

1. Dische, S., Saunders, M.I., Lee, M.E., Adams, G.E. and Flockhart, I.R. (1977) Br. J. Cancer, 35, 567-579.

2. Thomlinson, R.H., Dische, S., Gray, A.J. and Errington, L.M. (1976) Clin. Radiol., 27, 167-174.

3. Sealy, R. (1978) Br. J. Cancer, 37, Suppl. III, 314-317.

4. Watson, E.R., Halnan, K.E., Dische, S., Saunders, M.I., Cade, I.S. McEwen, J.B., Wiernik, G., Perrins, D.J.D. and Sutherland, I. (1978) Br. J. Radiology, 51, 879-887.

5. Dische, S. (1978) Br. J. Radiology, 51, 888-894.

6. Urtasun, R.C., Band, P., Chapman, J.D., Feldstein, M.L., Mielke, B. and Fryer, C. (1976) New Engl. J. Med. 294, 1364-1367.

7. Dische, S. (1974) Br. J. Radiol., 47, 99-107.

MISONIDAZOLE - A DRUG FOR USE IN ONCOLOGY

STANLEY DISCHE

Marie Curie Research Wing for Oncology, Regional Radiotherapy Centre,

Mount Vernon Hospital, Northwood, Middlesex, England

ABSTRACT

Misonidazole is an hypoxic cells radiosensitizer with promise in clinical radiotherapy. The concentrations which may be achieved in humans in serum, tumours and in all tissues are discussed. The toxic effects of misonidazole are detailed and schemes for the safe administration in man are described.

INTRODUCTION

In 1974, Ro-07-0582 (misonidazole), was shown to be an efficient radiosensitizer in animal tumours known to contain hypoxic cells. Clinical experience with this drug comprised only limited testing in humans as a possible trichomonaside in 1965 using low doses (Lenox-Smith, 1975[1]): it was effectively a new drug as opposed to metronidazole which had received extensive use as a trichomonaside though in rather lower dosage to that required for radiosensitization. In 1974 we administered the drug in doses of between 1-4 g to six normal volunteers (Foster, et al. 1975[2]). Permission was then granted to give the drug to a limited number of patients suffering from advanced malignant disease. In a series of eight patients given single doses between 4-10 g satisfactory serum concentrations were achieved similar to those seen in animals where radiosensitization had been clearly demonstrated (Gray, et al. 1976[3]). There were some gastro-intestinal disturbances, particularly in the patients given high doses, but otherwise in the single dose study tolerance was good. Promising results were obtained from studies of skin reaction in hypoxic skin and in the response of tumour in patients where multiple nodules were irradiated with or without the sensitizer (Dische, et al. 1976[4]; Thomlinson, et al. 1976[5]).

Encouraged by this study we moved on to give the drug in multiple doses to 16 patients. Unfortunately the drug proved to be neurotoxic, producing convulsions in the patients given the highest dose and peripheral neuropathy in another 11 where the dose was reduced (Dische, et al. 1977[6]). A further reduction in dosage was required and this has given a lower and acceptable incidence of peripheral neuropathy (Saunders, et al. 1978[7]; Dische, et al. 1978[8]). Reports upon the use of misonidazole have now been made by Urtasun, et al. 1977[9] and 1978[10]; Sealy, 1978[11]; Wiltshire et al. 1978[12]; Jentzsch, et al. 1977[13]; Kogelnik, et al. 1978[14] and Phillips, et al. 1978[15] recording the international experience of the drug in Canada, South Africa, Austria and the United States, as well as further experience in the United Kingdom. At Mount Vernon we have now extended our study to over 150 patients.

There has been considerable discussion as to the best method to employ the permitted dose of misonidazole. The drug can be administered in a few large doses combined with a large dose of radiation (Dische and Saunders, 1978[16]; Sealy, 1978[11]). Others give the drug in a similar fashion with treatments with misonidazole separated by smaller doses of radiation without the drug (Wiltshire, et al. 1978[12]; Kogelnik, et al. 1978[14] and Phillips, et al. 1978[15]). We have advocated the use of the drug combined with conventional daily fractionated radiotherapy as a method to be explored along with other schedules (Dische, et al. 1978[8]).

This paper describes the clinical experience of the use of misonidazole as regards its administration, plasma concentration, normal tissue and tumour concentration and toxicology.

METHODS

The patients studied were attending the Regional Radiotherapy Centre at Mount Vernon Hospital. They suffered a variety of malignant disorders but mainly carcinoma of the bronchus, breast, bladder, uterus and cervix. All plasma and tissue concentrations were determined in the Gray Laboratory.

The assay of plasma samples from patients receiving misonidazole in conjunction with radiotherapy at Mount Vernon has been undertaken using one of three techniques: polarography, gas liquid chromotography or high pressure liquid chromatography.

Normal values in man

Misonidazole is readily absorbed from the stomach and a peak level in the plasma is achieved normally between 1-2 hours after oral administration. After the peak there is a period of slow fall which extends to about 5 hours and this has been called the plateau period (Figure 1) strictly ('total nitroimidazole concentration')

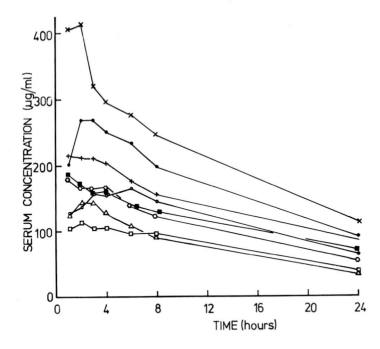

Fig. 1. When misonidazole is given to patients the blood concentration of drug rapidly rises to reach a peak in one to two hours. Commonly a plateau region is seen on the concentration curve at between $3\frac{1}{2}$ and $4\frac{1}{2}$ hours. (Gray, et al. 1976[3])

The total nitroimidazole concentration subsequently falls with a half-life of about 12 hours The mean plateau concentration achieved per gram of misonidazole given is 23.4 μg/ml. It can be seen from Table 1 that the variance is reduced by correcting for body weight and still further by correcting for surface area. This confirms the general use of surface area when calculating the dose for any one patient. We have found that the plateau concentration achieved per gram of misonidazole given is lower in men than in women but on the other hand the half-life of the drug in women is shorter than in man. These differences remain after correction for body size. It has been shown that there is a near-linear relationship between dose given and plasma concentration in both men and women.

TABLE 1

Half-life and plateau concentration of misonidazole in 130 patients

MALES				
Measurement	Mean	S. D.	Cases	OBS
Half-life	13. 22	2.91	71	156
Plasma conc /g misonidazole given	21. 28	4. 58	78	386
(Conc /g) (Wt /Mean Wt)	21. 22	4. 20	78	386
(Conc /g) (SA /Mean SA)	21. 33	4. 01	72	371
FEMALES				
Measurement				
Half-life	11. 56	3. 29	45	96
Plasma conc /g misonidazole given	26.99	6.11	52	230
(Conc /g) (Wt /Mean Wt)	26.92	6.65	52	230
(Conc /g) (SA /Mean SA)	26.99	6. 05	44	217
ALL CASES				
Measurement				
Half-life	12. 59	3.16	116	252
Plasma conc /g misonidazole given	23. 41	5. 89	130	616
(Conc /g) (Wt /Mean Wt)	23. 24	5.17	130	616
(Conc /g) (SA /Mean SA)	23. 28	4. 89	116	588

The values have been corrected for patient's size in each case by
multiplying by the patient's weight over the mean weight and by the
patient's surface area over the mean surface area.

The concentration in normal and tumour tissue

The first estimates of tumour concentration in man showed a wide range from
13-100% of the corresponding plasma concentration at time of estimate, (Gray, et al.
1976[3]).   Later studies using improved techniques for preparation of the specimens
have given values in excess of 40% and usually in the range of 60-100% (Dische, et al.
1977[6]). The inclusion of a small amount of normal fat in the specimen may
considerably lower the result because the partition co-efficient fat /water for
misonidazole is 1:3.

Similar tumour tissue values have been obtained by Urtasun, et al. 1977[9];
Dawes, et al. 1978[17]; Wiltshire, et al. 1978[12] and Ash, 1978[18]. Estimates of the
concentration of misonidazole in normal tissues have been performed by Urtasun, et al.
1977[9] and Ash, 1978[18], showing similar findings to those in tumour tissue.

Misonidazole levels rise rapidly after oral administration in the cerebro-spinal fluid (Urtasun, et al. 1977[9]; Wiltshire, et al. 1978[12]) with a peak concentration occurring soon after that in the plasma. Usually levels are nearly at the height of those in the plasma but some lower values have been recorded (Kogelnik, et al. 1978[14]; Ash, 1978[18]).

Metabolism of misonidazole

Studies have been performed in mice, rats, baboons and in man (Flockhart, et al. 1978[19]). There are large differences between men and the animals studied as regards the half-life of the drug in plasma: in the mouse this is between 1 and 1.5 hours, in the rat 1.7 hours and the baboon 4.5 to 5.5 hours compared with approximately 12 hours in man.

In all species examined small amounts of the breakdown product desmethylmisonidazole may be detected after 4 hours in the plasma but this rarely exceeds 20% of the misonidazole level. This compound is also active as a radiosensitizer. Approximately 10% of the drug is excreted in the urine within the first 24 hours as unchanged misonidazole and 8% as desmethylmisonidazole, but there is a wide variation. Further studies including the use of C-14 labelled misonidazole in man performed at Mount Vernon Hospital, in collaboration with Roche Products Ltd. have shown a continued excretion of drug unchanged and desmethylmisonidazole for at least 48 hours after administration and up to 50 or 60% may be accounted for by urinary excretion.

Extensive faecal excretion does not occur with this nitroimidazole in man in contrast to other species such as the mouse and with other nitroimidazoles given to man such as metronidazole. No loss in respired air has been found in either mice or man.

The remainder of the drug currently unaccounted for is, we believe, broken down by hepatic enzymes and excreted only slowly (Flockhart, et al. 1978 unpublished observation). There is no evidence for significant loss in other tissues.

Direct diffusion into tumours

The ability of misonidazole to diffuse deeply into tissues has led to attempts at direct diffusion of the drug into tumours. Awwad, et al. 1978[20] reported their findings following the introduction of misonidazole into the bladder 2 hours before cystectomy for carcinoma secondary to schistosomiasis. In five of seven cases concentrations of the order of 400 $\mu g/g$ were detected in tumour, but not in normal bladder tissues. We have repeated this work in five patients with carcinoma of bladder, two underwent cystectomy and three endoscopic biopsy. Although very high concentrations were achieved in one case, lesser levels were reached in others and the normal tissue concentrations reached considerable levels. Further work concerned with direct diffusion is proceeding.

Toxic effects

1. Gastro-intestinal disturbances Anorexia, nausea and vomiting were noted in our first group of patients who were given large single doses of the drug. This was certainly dose-related and was troublesome in those given the highest doses. These patients were all suffering from widespread malignant disease and were receiving considerable radiotherapy in association with the drug. Misonidazole was given these patients always on an empty stomach. A considerable bulk of material had to be given - up to 20 tablets either in their intact form or crushed and made into a suspension in fruit juice. The drug itself has an unpleasant taste and this has certainly contributed to anorexia and nausea. In subsequent work the patients have on the whole been fitter, the dose given has been smaller and capsules are now used. Further, patients have been allowed a light breakfast and the drug usually given at about 10 am. No gastro-intestinal disturbance of any significance has since been observed by us. Nausea and vomiting have been reported by other workers (Urtasun, et al. 1978[10]; Phillips, et al. 1978[15], Kogelnik, et al. 1978[14] and Sealy, 1978[11]) and also constipation (Sealy, 1978[11]).

2. Neurotoxic effects Convulsions have occurred in two of our patients, one given the largest dose (51 g in 6 fractions over 17 days) and also in another patient given two large doses totalling 16 g where the doses were separated by a period of three days. In the latter patient there was an unusually high serum concentration for the dose administered and a prolonged half-life. In both cases convulsions commenced at 20 hours after administration of the last dose, followed by considerable impairment of brain function which showed only a partial improvement before each of the patients died. Both were suffering from advanced malignant disease and death was primarily due to this though the neurological damage contributed (Dische, et al. 1977[6]; Saunders, et al. 1978[7]).

Peripheral neuropathy

In a series of 14 patients given misonidazole in 4,5,6 or 15 to 20 doses over a period of between 17 and 28 days and where the total dose given was approximately 15-16 g per square metre of surface area, 11 suffered peripheral neuropathy. This was of onset between 15-30 days after the beginning of treatment and in some caused the drug to be discontinued during the course of radiotherapy. It took the form of numbness and paraesthesia in the hands and feet with the most troublesome symptoms persistent in the feet. Some patients went on to suffer cramp-like pains in the feet extending up into the calves. Objectively sensory impairment to light touch and pinprick was observed in the toes in most of the patients and this extended up into the lower leg in some cases. Usually the symptoms gradually subsided after a period of several weeks, but in some they persisted until death and one patient remained troubled at two years. We have not been able to demonstrate any motor loss in our patients, but this has been reported by other workers (Phillips, et al. 1978. Awaiting publication[21]).

In our subsequent work a reduction of dose to 12 g per square metre of surface area given over a period of at least 17 days resulted in a reduction of peripheral neuropathy to 30%. With monitoring of the serum concentration and appropriate reduction of dose in some cases this has now been reduced to 12% and in nearly all the cases it is of such mild severity as to be of no great clinical importance.

It might be that a larger total dose can be given either when the period of treatment exceeds four weeks or when the drug is given in a single weekly dose. Further work is required to show whether this is so. A collaborative effort involving six centres where work with misonidazole is proceeding may, by pooling of data, lead to an early answer to this question (Dische, et al. 1978[22]).

Transient neurological disturbances

We have observed in five patients following one up to three administrations of misonidazole in large doses the appearance of a transient peripheral neuropathy which appears about 12 hours after administration of the drug and which disappears after about 24 hours. The symptoms do not occur with other identical doses given to the same patients. The appearance of this transient disturbance does not seem to be related to later occurrence of established peripheral neuropathy and seems of no clinical importance. We have in one patient observed a mild confusional state associated with transient changes in the plantar response and deep reflexes of the legs. In this patient a series of six doses of 3 g were planned over a period of 17 days and the confusional state appeared after the second dose. The drug was discontinued after the fourth when the patient made a gradual but complete return to normality over the subsequent 10 days. No other cause could be found for these symptoms and it seems likely that they were related to the administration of misonidazole.

Confusional disturbances are not uncommon in elderly patients with advanced neoplasms and if such patients are given misonidazole it is often difficult to determine if the drug is contributing. In only the one case described were we convinced that this was so, but this may have occurred in others. It appears, however, to be a relatively minor problem. Professor Sealy has reported a transient episode of ataxia in one of his patients and vertical mystagmus in another, but alcohol in excess may have been responsible in both cases. Jentzsch et al. 1977[13] have reported the appearance of a drug related organic psycho-syndrome but in both cases where this was observed all manifestations disappeared within one week. All these transient disturbances due to misonidazole seem to settle without leaving any persistent abnormality.

Skin rashes

Hypersensitivity skin rashes due to misonidazole have been recorded in three of our patients. A maculo-papular rash appeared between 8 and 17 days after beginning radiotherapy with misonidazole after a dose of between 6.5 and 7g of drug had been given. The maculo-papular rash appeared on the arms, hands, feet and legs and also on the trunk in two cases. In one, misonidazole was readministered and provoked recrudescence of the rash. In our three cases the rashes were not especially troublesome but did lead to the premature cessation of misonidazole administration. In four other cases rashes appeared, not dissimilar in type, during courses of radiotherapy with misonidazole but in all four the cautious re-administration of misonidazole did not provoke recrudescence of the rash and it was considered that the misonidazole may not have been responsible. A similar rash also appeared in one of the control cases in a clinical trial who was not given misonidazole.

Similar cases have been observed by Sealy in Capetown and Kogelnik in Vienna. All these cases have now been recorded (Saunders, et al. 1978[23]). Two further cases have been reported by Partington, et al. 1978. Awaiting publication[24].

Eighth nerve symptoms

Eighth nerve disturbances have been reported by Phillips, et al. 1978[15] and Kogelnik, et al. 1978[14]. These workers tend to use large doses on a weekly basis and this may account for the appearance of such symptoms in their patients, but not those treated at other centres. The symptoms are apparently transient and no permanent change results.

The plasma concentration measurements and misonidazole toxicity

It was shown in the first series of cases given multiple doses of misonidazole that the incidence of peripheral neuropathy was related to the tissue exposure as estimated from the curve of plasma concentration given after each dose of the drug (Dische, et al. 1976[4]). Further work has confirmed this observation. In a series of 43 patients planned for identical misonidazole therapy, six doses over 17-18 days, to a total of 12 g per square metre, those who suffered peripheral neuropathy showed significantly higher plateau values and tissue exposure as indicated by the product of the plasma concentration at the plateau period multiplied by the half-life (Table 2). We believe, therefore, that it is important to monitor the plasma concentration not only to pick up those few patients who show unusually high values and who must, therefore, be specially at risk for development of misonidazole toxicity, but also to pick up those who show values in the upper part of the normal range when a small reduction of misonidazole dose may appreciably reduce the risk of peripheral neuropathy. Because in any one patient fairly consistent readings are obtained through a course of treatment only a limited number of examinations is necessary.

The high plateau concentration seen in women is partly compensated for as regards tissue exposure by a shorter half-life. However, calculation of mean exposure indices show that for women to be 10% greater than that for men. We have not seen an overall increase in neurotoxicity in women compared with men but this may be related to differences in the numbers of men and women in the different dose groups. Among the 43 patients given six doses of misonidazole and referred to above there were only seven women, but four developed peripheral neuropathy compared with 10 of the 36 men.

TABLE 2

An analysis of the data concerning 43 patients planned for 6 treatments with misonidazole and radiotherapy using a total of 12 g per square metre of surface area. The patients have been divided into those free of peripheral neuropathy and those suffering from it. The mean of the plasma levels (at the plateau period) is significantly higher in those with neuropathy. The significance is increased when the half-life measurement is also taken into consideration and the exposure index calculated (plasma level x half-life)

	No Neuropathy			Neuropathy			Statistical Tests	
	Cases	Mean	Standard Deviation	Cases	Mean	Standard Deviation	Student 'T'	P
Age (years)	28	63.36	9.18	14	64.00	9.45	0.21	0.84
Height (m)	29	1.70	0.08	14	1.66	0.06	1.55	0.13
Weight (kg)	29	67.77	10.58	14	64.86	13.48	0.75	0.46
Dose (g)	29	18.40	2.59	14	17.82	2.72	0.65	0.52
Number of doses	29	5.93	0.25	14	5.86	0.35	0.77	0.45
Treatment time (days)	29	19.38	1.88	14	18.36	1.87	1.63	0.11
Surface area (m^2)	29	1.78	0.16	14	1.72	0.19	1.15	0.26
Average dose (g)	29	3.11	0.47	14	3.05	0.49	0.35	0.73
Dose /Weight (g /kg)	29	0.28	0.04	14	0.28	0.05	0.38	0.71
Dose /SA (g /m^2)	29	10.35	1.26	14	10.40	1.17	0.13	0.90
Mean Plasma Conc. μg /ml /	29	65.89	6.31	14	70.34	6.75	2.07	0.046
Mean T1 /2	29	12.40	2.56	12	13.77	2.07	1.60	0.12
'Exposure Index'	29	4849	1090	12	5701	1009	2.47	0.030

Dose regimes

Misonidazole is presently supplied by the Roche Company in capsules containing 500 mg and 100 mg. A scheme for administration of misonidazole has been devised based on the total allowed dose of 12 g per square metre of surface area and the strength of these preparations.

We often employ a six dose regime given twice weekly for three weeks. The plateau and 24 hour concentrations are determined after the first dose. If satisfactory we take plateau levels only at the second, fourth and sixth doses to monitor the course. If initial readings are above the line in Figure 2 we make appropriate reductions in dose. When misonidazole is given in six doses we normally use only the 500 mg capsules: we divide the permitted dose (12 g per square metre of surface area) by six and if the dose falls between half gram levels give the lower dose. If the plasma concentration permits we can later elevate the dose to the higher dose level.

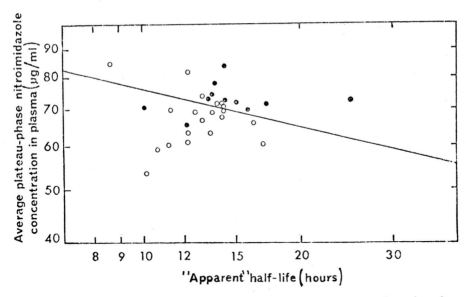

Fig. 2. Chart employed for adjustment of dose when patient given six doses based on a total of 12 g per square metre of surface area. The ● indicates a patient who developed neuropathy and ○ a patient who did not, using the same regime (Dische, et al. 1977[6]).

In daily treatments we have experience of over 60 patients where the drug was given on four of five working days each week. Until recently only 500 mg capsules or tablets have been available, but we were able to divide the tablets so as to give a unit of 250 mg. The plasma concentrations obtained in the plateau period are illustrated in two cases (Table 3). In Case 611 it was intended to give 20 doses of misonidazole with radiotherapy, treating on Mondays and Tuesdays and on Thursdays and Fridays over a period of five weeks. Because of a Public Holiday this scheme was altered in the second and third weeks.

TABLE 3

The plateau concentrations obtained in two patients through courses of radiotherapy with misonidazole

		Case 611 Ca. Bladder 20 doses 20g total	Male		Case 459 Ca. Breast 25 doses 19.5g total	Female	
	Week	Misonidazole g	Plasma Concentra- tion µg/ml	Week	Misonidazole g	Plasma Concentra- tion µg/ml	
	M				M		
	T				T		
1	W			1	W	1.0	24.5
	Th	1.0	16.5		Th	0.75	21.5
	F	1.0	20		F	0.75	22.5
	M	1.0	18		M	1.0	26
	T	1.0	25		T	0.75	26.5
2	W	1.0	21	2	W	0.75	24.5
	Th	1.0	20		Th	0.75	24.5
	F				F	0.75	22
	M				M	1.0	24
	T	1.0	15.5		T	0.75	24
3	W	1.0	21	3	W	0.75	21
	Th	1.0	20		Th	0.75	23.5
	F	1.0	20.5		F	0.75	22.5
	M	1.0	15		M	1.0	26.5
	T	1.0	19.5		T	0.75	22.5
4	W			4	W		
	Th	1.0	20		Th		
	F	1.0	23		F		
	M	1.0	16		M	0.75	17.5
	T	1.0	19		T	0.75	22
5	W			5	W	0.75	23.5
	Th	1.0	16		Th	0.75	24.5
	F	1.0	19.5		F	0.75	26
	M	1.0	15.5		M	0.75	20.5
	T	1.0	19.5		T	0.75	21
6	W			6	W	0.75	24.5
	Th				Th	0.75	19
	F				F	0.75	23.5

A uniform dose of one gram was given on each occasion. Because of the relatively long half-life of the drug some 10-30% of the plateau concentration remains at 24 hours. This means that in daily administration the dose on the second day will result in a higher level. This can be clearly seen in this patient. When the drug is continued on every day the concentration on the second and subsequent days tends to remain constant. In an effort to obtain uniform concentration at every treatment the dose on the first day can be increased. This is illustrated in the record obtained in case 459 (Table 3). The patient was treated for an advanced carcinoma of breast by radiotherapy given initially in a three week course to breast and glandular areas followed by a two week course where treatment was localised to the primary site. An elevation of the dose on the first day of treatment each week has resulted in a more constant level being obtained. This was not carried out in the last two weeks of treatment.

Although the adjustment of dose does give a more even concentration at time of treatment the variations are relatively small and sometimes may not be easily discernible among the variations which must be expected from day to day. We have concluded that the complications which may result from varying the dose due to confusion on the part of the patient do not make this variable dosage worthwhile and recommend a uniform dose throughout treatment. The following scheme based upon the 12 g per square metre of surface area is now being employed.

Misonidazole in radiotherapy using daily treatment

Calculate patient's surface area. Read daily dose from chart according to number of doses planned for patient

	Number of doses			Daily
	20	24	30	Dose mg
	2.0			1200
Surface	1.8			1100
area	1.7	2.0		1000
	1.5	1.8		900
Square	1.3	1.6	2.0	800
metres	1.2	1.4	1.8	700
		1.2	1.5	600
			1.3	500

Monitor the plasma concentration on first three days during plateau period ($3\frac{1}{2}$-$4\frac{1}{2}$ hours after administration when radiotherapy is given)

Plasma level should not exceed

Number of doses
20   24   30

Plasma concentration μg/ml
30   28   25

Proportional reductions should be made in daily dose if necessary when it would also be necessary to make further daily checks. Subsequently the plateau plasma concentration should be monitored once a week, preferably on a Thursday or Friday, in order to make certain that there is no accumulation of drug concentration. In our experience, however, such accumulations are very uncommon.

CONCLUSIONS

Misonidazole is the first hypoxic cell radiosensitizer showing considerable promise of benefit to arrive for use in the clinic. Unfortunately neurotoxicity limits the dose which may be employed. A maximum dose of 12 g per square metre of surface area seems to be safe provided that the drug is given over a period of 17 or more days. The demonstration of the cytotoxic effect independent of radiosensitization by this compound and others related to it suggests that the drug may have value in combination with cytotoxic agents in the cytotoxic chemotherapy of cancer (Hall and Biaglow, 1977[25]). This experience with regard to the administration of misonidazole in radiotherapy may, therefore, have an even wider application.

REFERENCES

1. Lenox-Smith, I. (1975) Personal communication.

2. Foster, J. L., Flockhart, I. R., Dische, S., Gray, A. J., Lenox-Smith, I. and Smithen, C. E. (1975) Br. J. Cancer, 31, 679-683.

3. Gray, A. J., Dische, S., Adams, G. E., Flockhart, I. R. and Foster, J. L. (1976) Clin. Radiol., 27, 151-157.

4. Dische, S., Gray, A. J. and Zanelli, G. D. (1976) Clin. Radiol., 27, 159-166.

5. Thomlinson, R. H., Dische, S., Gray, A. J. and Errington, L. M. (1976) Clin. Radiol., 27, 167-174.

6. Dische, S., Saunders, M. I., Lee, M. E., Adams, G. E. and Flockhart, I. R. (1977) Br. J. Cancer, 35, 567-579.

7. Saunders, M.I., Dische, S., Anderson, P. and Flockhart, I.R. (1978) Br. J. Cancer, 37, Suppl. III, 268-270.

8. Dische, S., Saunders, M.I. and Flockhart, I.R. (1978) Br. J. Cancer, 37, Suppl. III, 318-321.

9. Urtasun, R.C., Band, P.R., Chapman, J.D., Rabin, H., Wilson, A.F. and Fryer, C.G. (1977) Radiology, 122, 801-804.

10. Urtasun, R.C., Chapman, J.D., Feldstein, M.L., Band, R.P., Rabin, H.R., Wilson, A.F., Marynowski, B., Starreveld, E. and Shnitka, T. (1978) Br. J. Cancer, 37, Suppl. III, 271-275.

11. Sealy, R. (1978) Br. J. Cancer, 37, Suppl. III, 314-317.

12. Wiltshire, C.R., Workman, P., Watson, J.V. and Bleehen, N.M. (1978) Br. J. Cancer, 37, Suppl. III, 286-289.

13. Jentzsch, K., Karcher, K.H., Kogelnik, H.D., Maida, E., Mamoli, B., Wessely, P., Zaunbauer, F. and Nitsche, V. (1977) Strahlentherapie, 153, 825.

14. Kogelnik, H.D., Meyer, H.J., Jentzsch, K., Szepesi, T., Karcher, K.H., Maida, E., Mamoli, B., Wessely, P. and Zaunbauer, F. (1978) Br. J. Cancer, 37, Suppl. III, 281-285.

15. Phillips, T.L., Wasserman, T.H., Johnson, R.J., Gomer, C.J., Lawrence, G.A., Levine, M.L., Sadee, W., Penta, J.S. and Rubin, D.J. (1978) Br. J. Cancer, 37, Suppl. III, 276-280.

16. Dische, S. and Saunders, M.I. (1978) Br. J. Cancer, 37, Suppl. III, 311-313.

17. Dawes, P.J.D.K., Peckham, M.J. and Steel G.G. (1978) Br. J. Cancer, 37, Suppl. III, 290-296.

18. Ash, D. (1978) Personal communication.

19. Flockhart, I.R., Large, P., Troup, D., Malcolm, S.L. and Marten, T.R. (1978) Xenobiotica, 8, 97-105.

20. Awwaad, H.K., El-Merzabani, M.M. and Burgers, M.V. (1978) Br. J. Cancer, 37, Suppl. III, 297-298.

21. Phillips, T.L., Wasserman, T.H., Johnson, R.J., Gomer, M.S., Lawrence, G.A., Sadee, W., Marques, R.A., Levin, V.A. and VanRaalte, G. (1978) Int. J. Radiation Oncology Biol. Physics. Awaiting publication.

244

22. Dische, S., Saunders, M.I., Anderson, P., Urtasun, R.C., Kärcher, K.H., Kogelnik, H.D., Bleehen, N., Phillips, T.L. and Wasserman T.H. (1978) Br. J. Radiology (December 1978).

23. Saunders, M.I., Dische, S., Kogelnik, H.D. and Sealy, R. (1978) Awaiting publication.

24. Partington, J., Koziol, D., Chapman, D., Rabin, H. and Urtasun, R.C. (1978) Awaiting publication.

25. Hall, E.J. and Biaglow, J. (1977) Int. J. Radiat. Oncol. Biol. Phys., 2, 521-530.

Radiosensitizers of Hypoxic Cells
A. Breccia, C. Rimondi and G.E. Adams eds.

HYPOXIC CELL RADIOSENSITIZERS IN THE FUTURE DEVELOPMENT OF RADIOTHERAPY

G.E. ADAMS

Physics Division, Institute of Cancer Research, Clifton Avenue, Sutton, Surrey, England, SM2 5PX.

INTRODUCTION

The first lecture concluded with a brief introduction of the future prospects for misonidazole in clinical radiotherapy. This lecture proceeds from that standpoint and discusses first the limitations with existing drugs and suggests where future advances might possibly be made.

SOME PRESENT LIMITATIONS

a) Metronidazole: The weight of evidence from the laboratory indicates that the efficiency of metronidazole on a concentration basis might be of the order of 5-10 less than that of misonidazole. However, relative efficiency is less important than relative therapeutic ratio. If metronidazole were less toxic to man compared to misonidazole by an amount greater than the differences in the sensitizing efficiencies, then metronidazole would be the more effective drug, i.e. it would have a higher therapeutic ratio. However, the present indications are that although metronidazole appears to be somewhat less toxic than misonidazole in clinical use, this difference will probably not outweigh its reduced efficiency if the data obtained in experimental animal systems are a realistic guide. On present evidence then, misonidazole would appear to be the more effective drug, although considerably more clinical data would be required to finally prove the point. What is clear is that the doses of metronidazole that would be required to produce very large enhancement ratios in human tumours will not be attainable due to toxicity considerations.

b) Misonidazole: It is now apparent that the clinical dosage of this drug will be limited by its neurotoxicity although tolerated levels should be associated with a substantial degree of sensitization. Nevertheless, the maximum enhancement ratios for sensitization at the limit of dosage, irrespective of the administration schedule, will be significantly less than the theoretical maximum level of sensitization. While there is every encouragement therefore to pursue clinical evaluation of misonidazole as a sensitizer in radiotherapy, there is clearly a need to develop and investigate in the clinical, drugs of even higher therapeutic ratio. This aspect of the field is discussed later.

HOW SHOULD MISONIDAZOLE BE USED IN THE CLINIC?

Dische discusses, elsewhere in these Proceedings, the factors affecting the tolerance of this drug in man. On the evidence of the results of the Phase 1 clinical studies, it is recommended that the total clinical dose of misonidazole should not exceed 12 g/m^2. On this basis we can examine the maximum extent of sensitization that could be obtained theoretically, when misonidazole is used with different regimes employing fractionated radiothe rapy.

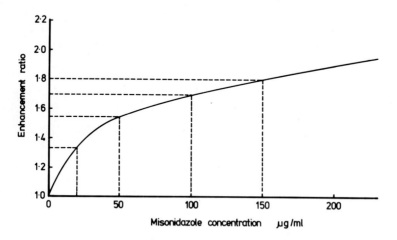

Fig. 1 - Dependence of enhancement ratio for irradiated Chinese hamster cells on misonidazole concentration.

Figure 1 reproduces the curve showing the dependence of the enhancement ratios for sensitization of hypoxic Chinese hamster cells on the concentration of misonidazole. It was stated earlier that the proposition that such a curve might apply to the sensitization of hypoxic cells in human tumours probably rests on two main assumption: 1) that the sensitization efficiency of misonidazole is not reduced for hypoxic cells *in vivo* compared to those *in vitro*; 2) the concentration of the drug achieved in hypoxic tumour cells approaches that in the serum. There is good evidence supporting both these assumptions.In the lecture by Dr. Fowler, results are given from several experiments with solid tumours in mice showing that the efficiency of misonidazole for sensitizing these tumours is as high as it is for the sensitization of hypoxic cells *in vitro*.

There is now considerable data on the penetration of misonidazole in human tumours obtained from analysis of surgical specimens. Occasionally, levels significantly lower than those measured in blood at the same time are observed. However, in many cases, tumour levels appear to approach blood levels. Significantly, in those regions of tumours where hypoxic cells are thought to occur,i.e. in, or around, necrotic areas, the levels are also generally high. We can then be reasonably confident in predicting that misonidazole will be fairly efficient in penetrating most large human tumours. We can examine, on the basis of these assumptions, the maximum sensitization factors that might be obtainable in a multi-fraction course of radiotherapy. The dotted lines in Fig. 1 give the enhancement ratios corresponding to concentrations of 20, 50, 100 and 150 μg/ml. These ratios are respectively 1.3, 1.55, 1.7 and 1.8. The enhancement ratios are all substantially less than the theoretical maximum of about 3, and in a multifraction course of radiotherapy the ratios may be reduced even further by reoxygenation of hypoxic cells occurring during the overall treatment. How then should misonidazole be used,bearing in mind the limitation of 12 g/m^2 as a maximum total dose?

Possible dosage schedules can be grouped into three broad classes, with the drug given: a) with every fraction of conventional radiotherapy, using say 20-30 fractions, or b) with every fraction of an unconventional regimen

using a limited number of say, 6-10 fractions, or c) with some *but not all*
fractions of either conventional or unconventional fractionation regimens.
The smaller the total number of fractions the greater is the amount of drug
that can be given with each fraction. For example, for a six-course treatment
extending over three weeks, $2g/m^2$ of misonidazole can be given with each of
the six fractions. Blood levels with this dosage are in the region of 60-
-70 μg/ml (see Dische, these Proceedings) and interpolation from Fig. 1 would
suggest that this concentration could be associated with an enhancement ratio
as high as 1.6 in a non-reoxygenating situation. Alternatively, if the drug
is given with each fraction of a more conventional regimen of between 20
and 30 fractions, maximum dosage of drug per fraction would be substantially
less. Blood levels in the region of 20-25 ug/ml are obtained under such
conditions (see Dische) and the anticipated enhancement ratios would be of
the order of 1.3. In animal experiments, where sensitization has been measured
for tumour levels of this order, enhancement ratios somewhat greater than
this have been measured (see Fowler). However, the point remains that the
maximum enhancement ratio per fraction will decrease as the number of
fractions increases.

This would appear to indicate one direction to follow in clinical studies
with this drug and some clinical trials are in progress, or planned, using
small numbers of large radiation fractions with the sensitizer given with
each fraction. Others are in progress, or planned, where the drug is to be
given with some but not all of the radiation fractions. However, at this
point in time it is important to keep all options open. Clinical trials
using misonidazole in a conventional daily fractionation scheme must remain
a high priority for several reasons. It has often been suggested from past
radiobiological experiments, that the oxygen effect is much reduced, or even
absent, for radiation doses of less than about 200 rads. However, the
results of the recently concluded MRC (UK) randomised trials of the use of
hyperbaric oxygen in the treatment of stage 3 carcinoma of the cervix (see
Dische, these Proceedings) have indicated highly significant benefit in
schedules using fraction sizes of the order of about 200 rads.

In addition there is a report[1] that Chinese hamster cells irradiated *in vitro* after prolonged contact with misonidazole, show a decreased shoulder in the radiation survival curve. If this is true *in vivo*, then the overall sensitization could be fairly large in a course of treatment employing a large number of radiation fractions.

A third factor to be considered, and one that might have considerable future implications for the treatment of cancer, is that associated with the property of differential hypoxic cytotoxicity shown by misonidazole and related compounds.

CYTOTOXIC EFFECTS ON HYPOXIC CELLS

In 1974 Sutherland and colleagues,[2] using a multicellular spheroid model system, showed that metronidazole was much more toxic to hypoxic cells compared with its toxicity to oxic cells. Subsequently, the effect was demonstrated on hypoxic cells in suspension culture for metronidazole, misonidazole and other nitro-containing sensitizing compounds[3-8].

In aerated cultures of Chinese hamster V-79 cells, the cells continue to grow in the presence of high concentrations of misonidazole, i.e. of the order of 2 millimolar (Fig. 2).

Figure 3 shows survival curves for hypoxic cells maintained for several hours in contact with misonidazole. The cells, after exposure, are aerated, washed free of the drug and tested for colony-forming ability. The data (Fig. 3) show that after an initial induction period of shoulder, where cell viability appears to be unchanged, the cells then show a sharp decline in survival as the contact time increases. The greater the concentration of the drug, the shorter is the shoulder period and the steeper the survival curve.

This cytotoxic action against hypoxic cells is shown by some other sensitizers of this type. The mechanism is believed to be associated with anaerobic metabolism of the drug which probably involves the sequential reduction of the nitro group. This process produces a cytotoxic substance which causes cell death. Whitmore and colleagues have obtained evidence[1] indicating that the mechanism involves a production of a substance which, once formed, can then kill both oxic and hypoxic cells. If this is correct then

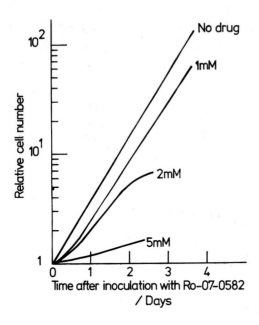

Fig. 2 - Growth of V78-378A Chinese hamster cells in suspension culture in air
in the presence of various concentrations of misonidazole at 37°C.
(ref. 7).

it represents a unique type of cytotoxic process.

There is sound evidence that the mechanism of this differential hypoxic
cytotoxicity is quite different from the mechanism of radiation sensitization.
Firstly, the data in Fig. 3 show that a prolonged contact time is necessary
for the cytotoxic effect to be manifest. In contrast, rapid mixing techniques[9]
have shown that hypoxic cells can be radiosensitized by drugs of this type,
including misonidazole, even though the pre-irradiation contact time is very
short, i.e. of the order of seconds or less. Secondly, the radiation
sensitizing ability of misonidazole appears to be unchanged over the temperature
range 0-37°C. In contrast, the hypoxic cytotoxic effect of misonidazole in
Chinese hamster cells in culture is highly temperature-dependent[6,7]. (See
lecture by Dr. Stratford,these Proceedings). This effect is also shown by
some other sensitizers. For example, the compound nitroimidazine, a 5-
-nitroimidazole, shows a temperature effect even more pronunced than
misonidazole[10]. Survival data at temperatures of 37, 39 and 41°C are shown
in Fig. 4.

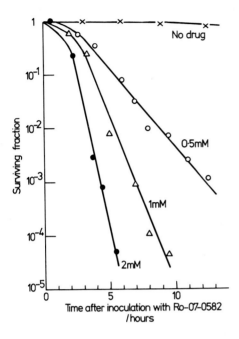

Fig. 3 - Survival of cells exposed to various concentrations of misonidazole under hypoxic conditions at 37°C. (ref. 7). X .... no drug; .... 0.5 mM; .... 1.0 mM; .... 2.0 mM.

There is clearly a pronounced temperature effect on the efficiency of the cytotoxic process which contrasts sharply with the lack of the temperature effect on the radiosensitizing ability of this drug. The two separate properties of misonidazole raise therefore the following question:

IS THE CYTOTOXIC EFFECT OF MISONIDAZOLE IMPORTANT IN RADIOTHERAPY?

Analysis of the dose-response relationship for the cytotoxic effect shows that the extent of cell killings is a function of both concentration and contact time. Hall and coworkers[11] have concluded on the basis of their data that the dependence of the cytotoxic effect on contact time is greater than its dependence on drug concentration. This has the following implication for misonidazole used as a radiosensitizer in radiotherapy. Although the sensitizing efficiency per individual fraction would be somewhat less in a conventional six weeks fractionation scheme relative to that in less conventional schemes employing a smaller number of fractions, the influence

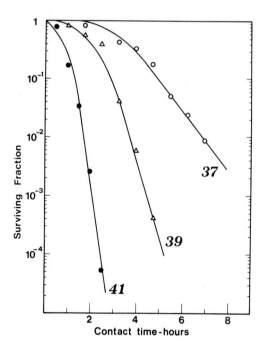

Fig. 4 - Effect of temperature on the cytotoxicity of 30 mM nitroimidazine
(a 5-nitroimidazole) towards hypoxic Chinese hamster cells (ref.10).

of the cytotoxic effect could be considerably greater. This is therefore an additional reason in favour of investigating the overall therapeutic benefits of misonidazole in the more conventional radiotherapy fraction regimens.

There is a real problem in investigating the cytotoxic properties of misonidazole in solid tumours in experimental mice. This is because of the relatively short half-life of the drug in these animals. As mentioned earlier, the half-life of misonidazole in mice is usually in the region of 1-2 hours contrasting with the much longer half-life of about 12 hours in humans. A further problem is that this short half-life, taken together with the time required for misonidazole to penetrate to hypoxic cells in solid tumours in mice, results in maximum tumour levels generally being considerably lower than the levels measured in blood. On the basis of the efficiency of the cytotoxic action measured in vitro, it has been calculated the even with a very large single dose administered to tumour-bearing mice, the degree of hypoxic cell kill would not be very large corresponding to a reduction of only one or two decades in cell survival. In contrast, the long half-life in humans indicates that even for quite low drug levels in human tumours the overall cytotoxic effect of misonidazole administered throughout a six weeks period, i.e. the time course for conventional radiotherapy, could be very considerable.

IS THE CYTOTOXIC EFFECT OF MISONIDAZOLE IMPORTANT IN CYTOTOXIC CHEMOTHERAPY?

The existence of the differential cytotoxic effect of misonidazole has a second implication with respect to cytotoxic chemotherapy. Chemotherapy is used widely in cancer treatment for the management of secondary metastatic disease. The possibility that hypoxic cells might constitute a relatively resistant sub-population of cells to the various cytotoxic agents has not been given the attention it warrants.

Various experiments with solid tumours in experimental mice have demonstrated that the efficacy of various cytotoxic agents is often reduced with increasing tumours size. An example of this is shown in Fig. 5 which reproduces data of Steel and colleagues,[12] for the treatment of an experimental mouse tumour X treated with the cytotoxic drug BCNU.

Mice were implanted with tumour cells in the thigh, and when the tumours had reached 0.5-1.0 cc in volume the animals were treated with BCNU. After sacrifice, the tumours were removed and the fraction of surviving clonogenic cells relative to those in control tumours, was measured by an *in vitro* method. The survival curve for tumour-bearing mice treated with various concentrations of this drug is shown in Fig. 5. Also shown in the Figure, is the survival curve for the response to BCNU of lung deposits of much smaller size. It is evident that BCNU is considerably more effective in the smaller tumours and this probably reflects the greater efficiency of penetration.

A second factor to be taken into account is that relatively small tumours can contain hypoxic cells, and if such cells are more resistant to various cytotoxic agents this could be an additional problem in the chemotherapy of metastatic disease. Shipley and co-workers have demonstrated[13] that Lewis lung tumours in experimental mice contain hypoxic cells when they exceed a total volume of about 15 mm^3. If hypoxic cells occur in small

254

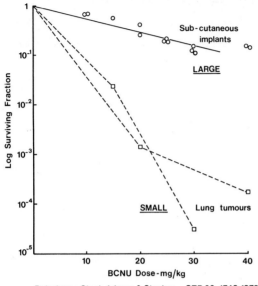

Fig. 5 - Cell survival after single doses of BCNU. The circles indicate
surviving fraction in large subcutaneous tumours. Square symbols
denote in two separate experiments surviving fraction on 1-2 mm
diameter lung colonies (see ref. 12).

human tumours then they would be a problem in the treatment of the tumours
by chemotherapy if these agents were indeed less effective in the absence
of oxygen.

Studies are being carried out in cells exposed *in vitro* to a variety of
cytotoxic agents under variable conditions of oxygen tension. Roizin-Towle
and Hall have noted that bleomycin in considerably less cytotoxic to hypoxic
Chinese hamster cells than it is in aerated suspension[14]. In our laboratory
we have observed similar behaviour with other cytotoxic agents. In particular,
data for the action of the drug actinomycin D on Chinese hamster V-79 cells
is given in Fig. 6.

Chinese hamster cells were exposed to a range of concentrations of this
drug for one hour. Cells exposed in hypoxia to the drug are substantially
more resistant than the aerated cells to the cytotoxic action of this drug.

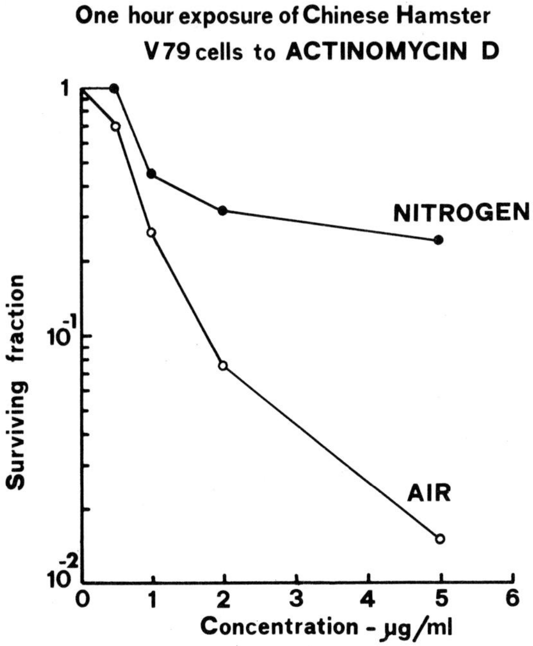

One hour exposure of Chinese Hamster
V79 cells to ACTINOMYCIN D

Fig. 6 - Survival curves for Chinese hamster cells treated for 1 hour with
Actinomycin D. O in air; ● in nitrogen.

In current work in our laboratory, we are finding that other drugs are less
effective cytotoxic agents to hypoxic cells compared with their effectiveness
against oxic cells. It is not yet known whether this relative resistance
will occur *in vivo*. However, this *in vitro* evidence, together with the
laboratory findings that tumour size is an important factor in the overall
effectiveness of some cytotoxic drugs, suggests that drugs that are
differentially toxic to hypoxic cells, e.g. misonidazole, may find a place
in combination-chemotherapy of malignant disease.

THE DEVELOPMENT OF NEW RADIOSENSITIZING DRUGS
    It is now clear that the toxicity of misonidazole will prevent it use
clinically at doses which will give the maximum theoretical level of
sensitization. There is, therefore, a need to develop new sensitizers with
better therapeutic indices. There are now hundreds of chemical compounds

now known which show appreciable sensitizing properties *in vitro* and there is no reason to suppose that the limit of efficiency *in vivo* has been attained with the only two drugs that have reached the clinical stage, i.e. metronidazole and misonidazole. Throughout the many years that the hypoxic sensitizer field has been developing, a wide range of active compounds have been found and this has been guided by various kinds of studies, both at the basic radiation chemical level and also in cellular systems. It is true that the requirements for sensitization of solid tumours *in vivo* disqualify many compounds that are otherwise very active as sensitizers *in vitro*. Nevertheless, structure activity studies using cellular systems *in vitro* have been most useful in establishing some of the guidelines for the development of new drugs.

It is now clear that the most important factor affecting sensitization efficiency is the electron affinity of the compound. This property is associated with the ability of a molecule to act as an oxidizing agent or electron sink at the radiation chemical level and is possessed by oxygen and many other chemical compounds. The higher the electron affinity of the compound, the greater is the sensitizing efficiency expressed in terms of the concentration required for a given amount of sensitization. In his lecture Dr. Wardman discusses in detail the background to the electron affinity correlation and discusses the methods used to establish structure activity relationships for drugs of this type. The data presented in Wardman's paper show that several compounds exist which are superior to misonidazole in sensitizing ability, again defined in terms of concentration required for a given degree of sensitization. However, in the search for new clinical sensitizers, data on the relative efficacies of different compounds are of limited value unless the appropriate information relevant to their toxic properties is also available. At the present time, one of the highest priorities is to obtain knowledge of the various structural, chemical, physical and biological characteristics of the sensitizers which might confer undesirable neurotoxic properties on these compounds.

Drug-induced damage to the peripheral nervous system in laboratory animals is susceptible to laboratory investigation and has been studied extensively for other types of drugs. Experiments have been performed on the effect of single doses of misonidazole on the conduction velocity in the sciatic nerves of treated mice[15] where there appears to be an acute depression of the velocity followed by rapid recovery after the drug has been cleared from the animal. Of possible significance also is the report[16] by Urtasun and colleagues of the occurrence of demyelination in peripheral nerve fibres of patients treated with misonidazole during radiotherapy. Behar, Liuni and Soffer[17] have shown that the antiseptic nitrofurantoin, which is also a radiosensitizer, causes demyelination in the sciatic nerve fibres in rats. However, much more work is required to establish the relevance of this phenomenon to the particular problem of the neurotoxicity of misonidazole in the clinical.

If it is true that demyelination phenomena are responsible for the neurotoxicity of sensitizers in man, then experimental studies will prove very useful as a prescreen for the study of the physical and chemical properties of sensitizers associated with the neurotoxicity. For example, if it transpired that demyelination is linked to the lipophilic properties of the sensitizers, this information would be most useful in the design of new drugs since lipophilicity does not appear greatly to affect sensitizing efficiency, at least *in vitro*.

REFERENCES

1. Whitmore, G.F., Gulyas, S. and Varghese, A.J. (1978) Brit. J. Cancer, 37, Supp. III, 115.

2. Sutherland, R.M. (1974) Cancer Res., 34, 3501.

3. Hall, E.J. and Roizin-Towle, L. (1975) Radiology, 117, 453.

4. Moore, B.A., Palcic, B. and Skarsgard, L.D. (1976) Radiat. Res., 67, 459.

5. Mohindra, J.K. and Rauth, A.M. (1976) Cancer Res., 36, 930.

6. Hall, E.J., Astor, M., Geard, G. and Biaglow, J. (1977) Brit. J. Cancer, 35, 809.

7. Stratford, I.J. and Adams, G.E. (1977) Brit. J. Cancer, 35, 307.

8. Numerous papers in "Hypoxic Cell Sensitizers in Radiobiology and Radiotherapy" (1978), Brit. J. Cancer, 37, Supp. III.

9. Adams, G.E., Michael, B.D., Asquith, J.C., Shenoy, M.A., Watts, M.E. and Whillans, D.W. (1975) in "Radiation Research: Biomedical, Chemical and Physical Perspectives", Nygaard, O.F., Adler, H.I. and Sinclair, W.K.

eds., Academic Press, p. 773.

10. Stratford, I.J., Watts, M.E. and Adams, G.E. (1978) in "Cancer Therapy by Hyperthermia and Radiation", Streffer, c. ed., Urban & Schwarzenberg, Baltimore-Munich, p. 267.

11. Hall, E.J., Miller, R., Astor, M. and Rini, F. (1978) Brit. J. Cancer, 37, Supp.III, 120.

12. Steel, G.G., Adams, K. and Stanley, J.A. (1976) Cancer Treatment Rep. 60, 1743.

13. Shipley, W.V., Stanley, J.A. and Steel, G.G. (1975) Cancer Res. 35, 2488.

14. Roizin-Towle, L. and Hall, E.J. (1978) Brit. J. Cancer, 37, 254.

15. Hirst, D.G., Vojnovic, B., Stratford, I.J. and Travis, E.L. (1978) Brit. J. Cancer, 37, Supp.III, 237.

16. Urtasun, R.C., Chapman, J.D., Feldstein, M.L., Band, R.P., Rabin, H.R., Wilson, A.F., Marynowski, B., Starreveld, E. and Shnitka, T. (1978) Brit. J. Cancer 37, supp.III, 271.

17. Behar, A.J., Livni, L. and Soffer, D. (1977) in "Neurotoxicology", Roizin, L., Shiraki, H. and Greevic, N. eds., Raven Press, New York.